Learn 2 Lose™

CW01647245

Copyright © 2024 Sophie Burr
All rights reserved.

ISBN: 978-1-06864-781-9 (paperback)

Learn2lose™ The information in this book is trademark-protected and must not be copied or reproduced.

SOPHIE BURR

Learn 2 Lose

transform your body and spread your wings.

"Without change, there would be no butterflies".

Contents

Dedication

I dedicate this book to my dad, who inspires me daily to pursue my dreams. He was never scared to take a chance on anything in life. Sadly, he was taken way before his time at the young age of just 68.

He was diagnosed with Type 2 Diabetes at the age of 40. Time eventually allowed this disease and all its complications to consume his body, and he could fight no longer.

I hope he is proud of me; he watches over me, keeps me safe and well, and pushes me to strive for more incredible things.

Sadly, the things I will share in this book could have saved my dad.

Everything happens for a reason, and his passing has led me to where I am now. Thank you, Dad, we miss you every day.

Disclaimer

I am not a medical doctor, and this book does not provide professional medical advice. It's essential to seek professional medical advice before starting any new nutrition-based plan.

One Size Does Not Fit All!

Please do not stop taking prescribed medication without first consulting your medical practitioner.

The advice in this book is a starting point for your very own Study of 1; remember: - One size does not fit all!

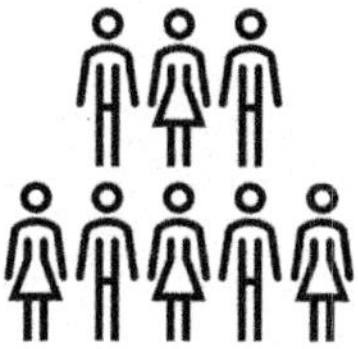

Acknowledgements

During this transformative journey of writing, there were moments when the path seemed daunting and the destination uncertain. Yet, it was in these moments of doubt that the true power of community revealed itself.

To my beloved Learn 2 Lose community, your unwavering belief in me illuminated the darkest of hours and fuelled the flame of determination within my soul. Pete, Daisy, Caitlin, and my dear mother, your unwavering support and attentive ears have been the pillars upon which I leaned during the toughest of times.

To my cherished friend who walked beside me on this path, your presence infused me with strength when my own faltered. You brought a unique perspective and a dose of encouragement that helped carry me through the challenges.

And to my late father, whose legacy of daring to defy convention and embrace change continues to inspire me daily. His spirit guides me as I aspire to challenge the norms of our medical landscape, advocating for a paradigm shift in how we are treated and perceived.

Let us remain steadfast in our resolve to champion new ideas and embrace a brighter tomorrow. We only pave the way for transformative change by daring to challenge the status quo.

With boundless gratitude and a heart full of hope,
Sophie xx

Introduction

In February 2019, I started writing while staying at my friend's farmhouse in northern France, in my pyjamas. Looking back, it's hard to believe what was going to happen. Nobody could have prepared us for the year that was to follow. And the reason it's taken me so long to finish this book.

In March 2020, the world came to a halt. We were instructed to keep our children at home, shut our doors, and stand 2 meters apart wearing a surgical mask. Airplanes were grounded, and we could hear birds singing.

COVID-19 affected each of us in different ways. Some lost loved ones and were unable to say goodbye, others had to keep their newborn babies away from cuddles with family, and some had to cancel their weddings multiple times. Everyone has their own personal pandemic story to share.

This was an opportunity to do what I love best: sit back and observe people. It never ceases to amaze me how humans behave when faced with adversity. This social experiment highlighted humanity's resilience and how kind and caring we can be to each other when faced with a real-life crisis.

Sadly, in 2024, we are now paying the price for drinking our body weight in Gin and becoming the best home bakers and fudge makers! The supermarkets were stripped of every snack we could find, and our carbohydrate addiction reached a whole new level!

As you read through the book, I know you will be able to relate specific chapters to the behaviours you have witnessed over the last couple of years. You will properly understand how our built-in survival mechanisms influence our decision-making and affect us mentally and physically.

We have now emerged from what we refer to as the great lockdown of 2020, and many of us came out the other side with a few more pounds to lose, and GPs are diagnosing thousands of people with type 2 diabetes. Suicide rates have hit an all-time high, and the economy is struggling to bounce back. Wow, that all sounds doom and gloom.

I firmly believe that everything happens for a reason and that we should throw things out to the universe to see what we get back. This book is designed to make you think and give you enough confidence to challenge people when they tell you how to lose weight.

I hope you enjoy the journey.

1

Where the story began

I want to start by telling you my story of how and why I am putting this all down on paper and sharing what I have learned.

My childhood was normal: mum, dad, and one older brother; we grew up in a small village in Kent. From a very young age, food was everything but ordinary to me. I must have been my mother's worst nightmare when it came to dinner time; I remember having a phobia of food from about 5. It physically scared me to touch, smell, or even get close to certain foods. There is now an actual diagnosis for this, known as ARFID (avoidant/restrictive food intake disorder). I remember starting primary school; my mum thought it would help me to try school dinner! Nope, big mistake! She wrote a letter to the school cook and sent me to hand it in.

I was happy that this would work; as a child, a letter from Mum meant they had to take notice, right? Sadly, no..

> ***"Sophie does not like certain foods so can she please be excused from what she does not like and just have what she does like to encourage her to try more foods".***

The evil school cook would let me choose three things I could decline, and the rest would be on my plate If I liked it! or not! So, in comes the role of the even more evil dinner ladies standing over me every day, watching me physically heave at the thought of lumpy mashed potato and fish pie that looked like it came from no fish I have ever seen! This continued for several weeks, and I was not allowed out to play and sat in the main hall at the last table, standing with one single chair, crying every lunchtime until it was time to return to class, and they couldn't legally keep me there any longer.

> ***"Why did I not tell my mum? I hear you ask".***

Sitting here writing this 42 years later, I still wonder the same myself! Luckily, my brother was two years ahead of me at the same school. Eventually, he ended my misery by telling my mum what they were doing to me every day, and I was released from any more childhood trauma and despatched into the packed lunch classroom the very next day.

Relieved to be in packed lunches, this brought a new world of issues! What the heck was she going to give me when I would hardly eat anything? Bear in mind that this was the early 80s, and the whole margarine phenomenon was sweeping the nation; my mum discovered that I would eat this weird stuff called St Ivel Gold, the thought of eating it now makes me feel almost as sick as the lumpy mash and fish pie! This was the era of my St Ivel Gold sandwiches phase, just as it sounds: bread with some plastic-tasting margarine-type stuff. I can't remember eating much else during those years except for one exception, potentially a rapid and easy bonus at mealtimes for my mum. My brother and I loved mince and Smash. Yes, she just had to add water and stir! My mum is a fantastic cook. I can't imagine now how she must have felt feeding me all these Franken Foods (fake foods made by Frankenstein).

It seems funny talking about it now, but this bizarre phobia of food stayed with me for many years and had a massive impact on going to play at friends' houses or eating out at restaurants right through to my late teens.

I can remember a little breakthrough for Mum. We went on holiday to St. Tropez and stayed on a campsite with a greasy chip van in the middle; I was brave and decided to try new food. I tried a chip, and I liked it. It was something new I would eat, Mum thought! But no, I told you it was a strange phobia! I would only eat St. Tropez chips, not chips made in Kent, as they wouldn't taste the same. It sounds bizarre, and I can imagine being so frustrated with my kids if they were to say something like this to me now, but to me, this was real; I believed actual physical harm was going to come to me with these foods.

So fast forward several weird eating years to the age of 16. This was the start of my dieting history. My mum, Nan, and friends were attending a slimming club to lose weight. Slimming Magazine Club was the name of it. It was held in our local leisure centre, and women flocked in to be told how good or bad they had been that week. I can remember the woman who ran the group. Her name was Pauline; she was tall, slim, blonde, and spiteful! You had to sign an agreement to say you would lose at least 5 lbs each month; otherwise, she would not allow you to come anymore!

This was enough of a threat to me to make me follow whatever evil Pauline said so I didn't get chucked out for poor performance. I only wanted to lose a stone, which now seems quite hilarious. I was 11 stone, and I wanted to be ten stone again; why is that magic 10-stone number so crucial to so many people? I do not know, but it was essential to me. I had recently started playing in an adult netball team, and they were all smaller than me. I wanted to order a 26-inch waist skirt like the others. OMG, 26 INCH! Yes, I once had a teeny tiny waist!

Unbeknown to me at the time, Slimming Magazine Club was a form of extreme calorie restriction; you got given these diet sheets each week where you could pick one thing from each box that had to be accurately weighed and measured, and the world would blow up if you cheated! The best one she gave me was the chocolate lovers' diet sheet, allowing me to choose a bite-sized chocolate bar daily.

Thinking back on this group, I realise it was the start of my 25 years or more of Yoyo dieting. I had swopped my very unhealthy childhood food phobia to a very restrictive diet culture. If only I could tell my 16-year-old self not to follow this broken path.

Fast-forward several more years to age 20, I met my now-husband Pete, and we moved into our first home together; this was a massive turning point for me when trying new foods. I was cooking for myself for the first time in my life, and that inspired me to expand my list of foods I ate from about 10 to maybe 20; it was still inferior, but I could handle a mushroom and some tomato puree or cheese if they were cooked or melted.

The biggest battle I now faced was Pete had two small boys that I was directly responsible for feeding at weekends;

I was conscious I did not want them to grow up with the same food phobias that had plagued my childhood, so I tried hard to make them try new foods, but I could not make them eat anything I didn't like myself, thankfully they turned out pretty standard, and now feed their little people.

During my early 20s, I gained and lost the same two stones a few times with various diets. Rosemary Conley was the main one of this era; fat was now the enemy in the 90s. I spent my life looking for foods with less than 5% fat per 100g, thinking if I just ate wine gums, that would be the answer! Rosemary Conley had a short 45-minute exercise class with the group, so this 45 minutes a week would save me from eating in the pub every night. My mum and I would go to the class and meet my dad and my husband Pete in the pub for dinner, undoing all the good we had just done; we may as well have set light to the £5 it had just cost us to be told we hadn't lost any weight.

I fell pregnant with my eldest daughter, Daisy, who was born in 2000; during my pregnancy, I felt sick almost every single day, and at 20 weeks, I discovered I had developed Gestational diabetes; this was a big concern for me as my Nan on my dad's side had died at age 58 from type 1 diabetes-related illnesses and my dad was also diagnosed at age 40 with Type 2. I had to test my blood glucose every time I ate; my finger was like a pin cushion! This helped me during my pregnancy as I did not gain lots of weight through fear of the condition developing further once the baby was born. Luckily, the diabetes disappeared shortly after her birth; by some freak of nature, I had only gained a stone in weight during the pregnancy, and I lost it the night she popped into the world. Miracle or what?

Little did I know that this was potentially a pivotal time in my life, leading to many years of Yo-Yo dieting.

So new baby, two minor stepchildren, running a stupidly busy cleaning business with my husband and working horrible unsocial hours, and not a great cook, this starts the takeaway crap food era of the new millennium, and on goes three stone without me even really noticing until perhaps when the clothes had jumped up three sizes and even my shoes didn't fit.

This started the Weight Watchers phase of my dieting history; Mum and Nan were going to a group again, so I tagged along. The lady who ran the group was called Lesley. She was lovely, and she is the person who inspired me most to want to help people to lose weight. Lesley was funny, inspiring, and, most of all, very typical. She had struggled all her life with weight problems, and she understood how we all felt; she didn't preach, she made the group fun, and I enjoyed going.

I lost three stone and was down to 11 again; I hadn't been this weight for many years. Mum and Nan also reached their goal weights, and the local paper even interviewed us for an article on three generations of one family losing weight at a local group. I also had a call from Weight Watchers media to feature on their website; I thought this would be a fantastic glamourous day of having my hair and makeup done and choosing some pretty clothes, but in reality, it was a nasty lock up in the depths of London somewhere really scummy with a tacky clothes rail. My hair and makeup were chucked together to make me look like someone who wasn't me! But I did get to keep the photos, at least!

So obviously, I thought I had cracked it now; I could follow Weight Watchers, Pro Points for the rest of my life, and the weight would stay off. It was going to be that easy.

Well, you've guessed it, the weight started coming back on; Lesley had left the group to go and be a landlady of a local pub as she couldn't adhere to the strict rules that Weight Watchers leaders had to stick to and stay within a healthy weight range, she shared with me in confidence, that they had to be weighed at a humiliating monthly meeting in front of all of the other leaders. She couldn't return to the range and felt she had to leave. This made me sad as I couldn't help but wonder why she didn't lose weight following the plan.

So, the weight started coming back slowly, but surely, 1 pound at a time, despite still following the plan at home. Aha, I thought, I need to be weighed on the magic scales in a group that will help me return to Target again.

A new Weight Watchers group was opening up in my local village hall. It must be fate, I thought, so off I went again, obviously knowing all the answers. The new lady was lovely, but she was no Lesley, and I kept paying each week and queuing up in the line to pay for £20 worth of Weight Watchers chocolate bars, crisps and gummy sweets that were nutritious and would help me lose weight! I swear the table with products was now four trestle tables long, and the talk got shorter and shorter while we waited for everyone to buy their weekly fill of Franken foods.

The icing on the Weight Watchers' cake for me came when I had saved up and treated myself to the crème de la crème of products, the magic food weighing scales that converted your food into points for you; how could I fail now with this item of pure genius! The following week, our leader, whom I can't even remember the name of (she was that good!), announced to the group that the plan was now changing to a new plan known as Pro Points; overnight, my new shiny £40 scales were worthless. The 58 cookery books I had acquired and never used were also useless! My mum and I stayed a few more weeks and decided we didn't like being deceived by the company or the leader with all the products we had purchased, and we decided to continue to follow the old plan ourselves at home.

Oh yes, you've guessed it. That didn't work either, and now two of the three stones are back again; I always seemed to bounce back to 13 Stone. I know this doesn't seem significant to many people, but to me, it felt massive, and I now had no clothes to fit again.

So, the following diet phase that hit my life was significant. Pete's brother and his wife called us and told us they had just what we had been looking for: a fantastic product to help us lose weight and a business all rolled into one; this was my introduction to Herbalife. This was the answer to all my prayers: you made two milkshakes a day from a range of flavours, vanilla, chocolate, strawberry or tropical, you drank some magic tea and your body weight in water and took a lot of magical vitamins that made me pee lots of smelly pee, and you had a typical meal in the evening. I lost weight initially, and Pete still swears by the Herbalife products to this day; I remain a distributor as it saves me money by keeping him supplied with his lemon thermo beverage that he would die without.

I tried and tried to make this work for me, but the old feelings of wanting to vomit at the primary school lumpy mash just came flooding back every time I took a sip of a milkshake. I tried it with apple juice, soya milk, skimmed milk, water, and yoghurt, but I couldn't find one I liked and could keep up with long-term. Plus, there was no way I was going out for lunch and taking a milkshake with me. This was the panini and latte decade!

I spent several years playing around with the products and even worked in a local gym for about four years, promoting them to the members as a wellness coach. We also travelled to many different places worldwide, listening to top nutritionists when they launched a new product; this part was probably the best as it sparked my love of nutrition. We met so many lovely people, but I wanted to know why the products worked and how they worked; I soaked up all the science I could lay my hands on. I couldn't make them work for me for sustained weight loss.

Herbalife is still strong today, and I know they have a vast Sports Nutrition following. Many friends make a great living by devoting their lives to the company and its enormous range of nutrition products.

It's now 2008, and yes, the same three stones are back, but there's a bigger shock: I'm pregnant. OMG, how did that happen? They never did find the missing coil (overshare, sorry).

So again, I'm feeling sick as a pig. I started losing weight as I couldn't eat very much, but my god, I could eat chocolate; I was waiting for them to say I had gestational diabetes again to stop the chocolate monster inside me! But weirdly, it didn't happen this time; this was a relief but also possibly a curse as I just munched my way through 9 miserable months of not wanting to be pregnant and feeling sick and feeding my face with Cadbury's. January 2009 came the birth of Caitlin, and by some freak of nature, the same thing happened; I had only gained one stone and lost it again overnight when she was born. How did that happen? I ate my body weight in chocolate and seemingly got away with it.

So, new baby, I've given up my job at the gym. I have an actual chocolate addiction; yes, the three stones I typically gain are now becoming four stones. I hit my all-time highest weight in 2010 of 14 stone 8, and my sister-in-law, who I worked for then, decided to join Slimming World. She is raving about the new fantastic plan called Extra Easy.

My eldest daughter, Daisy, had struggled with her weight since she was little and was always three sizes above the average for her age. I looked at the Slimming World website, and it said children could go if they were 11; she always looked much older than she was, so I thought we could get away with lying about her age, and she joined with me at age 10! Under a false Date of birth!

The Consultant Amanda was a bit scary on the first night as we arrived late. My sister-in-law told us it was 5.30 instead of 5.15, so we had to wait for the next new member talk at 7.15. By the time we finished, we were starving and bought a takeaway on the way home.

I liked the plan. It was pretty easy to follow, but I still didn't eat much fruit or vegetables, and Amanda kept raving about the magic speed foods you had to eat, which, in my world, would never happen. I desperately wanted to be able to wear the skinny jeans and long boots that Amanda wore to the group each week; they were my inspiration that a fat person could become a thin person, as she had lost over seven stone on this plan. I filled up on bucket loads of rice and pasta until my stomach hurt, but I was losing weight. I got my 2.5 stone certificate and shiny sticker and was so chuffed.

On the other hand, Daisy was following this plan, and she was getting bigger by the day; she would have a slight loss, and a significant gain would promptly follow it; it was heartbreaking. I knew she wanted to lose if only to keep me happy.

Shortly after getting my 2.5-stone shiny sticker, my dad fell very ill after major heart surgery; I have no idea how he survived. Still, by some miracle, he managed to fight back from 7 cardiac arrests and total organ failure after several weeks of hospital visits around the clock and living on Marks and Spencer's Yum Yums as a staple diet; I finally made it back to my slimming world group. I had gained pretty much everything I had lost in 3 short months. I was gutted, and Daisy had also gained at least another stone.

I managed to get back to 2 stone lost and got my 10 per cent award again, which meant I got a free week from the company, and they sent me a letter to ask if I would like to find out about becoming a consultant for Slimming World. This excited me, and I filled in the enquiry form and sent it back to the district manager, a lovely lady called Suzy. To my surprise, Suzy called me and invited me to an opportunity presentation to introduce the company and explain how the franchise worked. I went for an interview, and to my shock, I was turned down! I was gutted; I wanted to follow this dream. I persisted with Suzy, blagged another interview, and succeeded the second time. I paid £2000 for my franchise, and I was a fully-fledged Slimming World business owner.

I wholeheartedly believed in this plan, and I had very successful groups in a small town called Faversham; it made my heart skip when I saw the joy on people's faces when they received an award from me, but all the while, my daughter was still struggling. Her weight was increasing year after year. Some weeks, I would help up to 500 people in my five groups. It was mental, but for everyone I was helping, another one wasn't walking back in the door as they couldn't stick to the plan, or they went on holiday, had a significant gain, and couldn't face the scales.

In November of 2017, my dad sadly passed away after a very long battle with heart disease; it was finally acute Kidney failure and heart failure that took him from us; he was the biggest fan in my group. He came to my 7.30 session to weigh every single week and would always take my money home for me so I didn't get robbed on the way home; he never lost any weight despite my mum cooking all slimming world, world-friendly meals and making sure he had plenty of fresh fruit and veg and only ate low fat and sugar-free everything, in theory, it should have fallen off of him, but sadly it never did.

Dad wasn't alone; I had many friends in the group who were struggling, and I didn't have the answers to help them. In my head, I thought they must not be following the plan; that's why they were not losing weight, but I trusted these people in my heart. They had become my friends, and I wanted so badly to help them, but I didn't know how anymore.

After losing Dad, my weight ballooned again back up to 14 stone; I felt like a fraud standing in group week after week, telling people how easy this plan was and that I was struggling to follow myself! I couldn't do it anymore, and my grief was consuming me. My eating habits were getting worse by the day. I didn't want to diet anymore, and I had completely lost my passion for helping people lose weight, which saddened me deeply. The trouble was this was my life, job, and income. It put food on the table and paid the bills; I couldn't just walk away.

Daisy had been referred several years earlier to a dietician and paediatrician at the hospital. However, her weight was increasing year after year to the point where she was referred for gastric surgery at Kings College.

These were shallow points for me. I had failed to help my dad and my daughter, and now my younger daughter's weight was increasing to a dangerous level; she, too, was referred to the same paediatrician. Sadly, the Dr could not help us, but she did some more in-depth testing, and

"I don't buy junk food, we hardly ever eat take away foods, they eat fruit we have home cooked slimming world meals,"

we uncovered some actual medical issues with the girls that, at the time, I didn't realise how significant these would be in my quest to find a solution.

Every one of those appointments felt like it was all my fault; what had I done wrong? I can't tell you how many drunken conversations about the girl's weight had ended in me sobbing (I'm a very ugly crier!).

I felt like I was on trial. How can this woman help so many people lose weight, but she can't help those closest to her?

I swear my kids will be in therapy for years, blaming me for a lifetime of making them have such a bad relationship with food. I would find packets upon packets of sweets, crisps, and chocolate hidden in the weirdest places around the house; it was heartbreaking; the more I tried to restrict them to protect them, the worse the secret eating would get.

I was in such a desperate place with my group, my weight, and my daughter's weight, and I was desperately trying to come to terms with losing Dad; I didn't know what way to turn next. Weirdly, out of the blue, I had a phone call from a recruitment agency. He was a lovely, friendly man called Lawrence, and he started chatting about a post he was trying to fill, which he felt would suit a weight loss consultant. The position was working on the National Diabetes Prevention Programme, running small local groups for people at risk of Type 2 Diabetes; I listened and thought it was meant to be. I gave him my details and applied for the job. Lawrence phoned me a week later and said I didn't get an interview. I was gutted; at this point, I had given up 2 of my groups and was at rock bottom, just about managing to turn up each week and put a smile on my face.

A few months later, Lawrence phones again and says they are looking for someone else. This time, I made it to the interview and got the job. I handed in my notice to Slimming World, which was very sad after six years, and I made many friends along the way.

I felt like this position was made to help me give something back and not make Dads passing have been in vain. I was able to talk about him and my other family, who had suffered from the disease every day at work, and I struck a chord with people. I taught them how important it was to make the necessary changes to prevent this awful disease.

I was happy with my work, but sadly, I was still very unhappy with my weight; I could not get my dieting mojo back. I tried some Herbalife shakes again; they had a new flavour, "cookies and cream." I could tolerate it with skimmed milk, but no weight was lost. I even gained weight; I think I had a lactose overload at one point. I tried some funny pills and patches I bought from a woman online. All that did was hurt when I ripped the patch off, and still no weight loss. I also purchased the XLS medical pills they promote on the TV that are supposed to bind the fat in your food and make you lose more weight; they are still sitting on the desk in my office, and I kept forgetting even to take them!

In April 2019, my friend Sallyann messaged me to say she was unhappy with her weight and, like me, she has a huge family history of type 2 diabetes. Sal had lost weight with me at the gym with Herbalife and again at Slimming World and even became a consultant herself for a short while; she convinced me to brave it back to Slimming World as we both thought that was our most successful diet. Still, we just needed the group and a bit of moral support from each other, so off we went to my old group; I did get my half-stone certificate after about six weeks. Still, I couldn't sit in my old group and not be the one helping people, and neither could Sal; we agreed to meet at my house every

Wednesday for a weigh and measure, and we would do it on our own at home as nobody knew the plan better than us.

We both struggled to lose a couple more pounds and just gave up despite our best efforts, but we did enjoy a gin and tonic on a Wednesday after depressing ourselves that we still hadn't lost any weight! Why could we not lose? We followed the plan; Daisy also decided to be brave enough to join us. She was now at her heaviest weight of way over 20 stones and waiting to be given a date for her Gastric Sleeve Surgery.

It was summer 2019, and I was desperately trying to find some clothes to take on my summer holiday; we were going on a camping tour of France with my Favourite Cousin Lisa and her family; we named it *"Fat Chads on Tour"* (Chad is slang for bottom) her dad is my dad's brother and he was diagnosed with type 1 diabetes at the age of 11 and sadly lost his leg via amputation a few years previous so she like me has always known the importance of us keeping our weight in check and having a healthy diet.

We had a lovely holiday, and despite quite a lot of wine, we ate good food that we cooked ourselves every day and didn't overindulge, but still, the weight piled on; I had now hit 15.7, which was my heaviest weight by far ever!

Despite being desperately unhappy with my weight and avoiding looking at any holiday pictures, I was still more concerned about helping the girls as that August; I had to buy a size 20 ladies' trousers for Caitlin to go back to school at age ten she pretty much weighed the same as me at this point, buying school uniform for a 10-year-old girl that is the size of a fully grown woman made me feel physically sick, it is a pretty impossible task as they do not make ladies clothes that look like school uniform, anyone that has gone through the trauma of finding school uniform for a child that is not a uniform size or shape will feel this pain! No matter what we tried, we needed something to work for them. I just wanted to cry; why did we all struggle so much? was the constant dialogue in my head. I knew in my heart of hearts it wasn't about the food. I had so many arguments with my Nan, saying it must be what you feed them when they are with you, as this was the only explanation I could find, but they didn't spend that much time at my Nans, so I knew that couldn't be the real issue. People thought they were being kind, offering me advice, but it was nothing that I hadn't already tried. It was hopeless.

I sat down with my cousin Lisa, my friend Sal, and probably another ten telephone conversations with a close friend who was also my ex-slimming world consultant and said: -

"I am so desperate to lose weight,
but I just don't want to diet
anymore how can I do that?"

They thought I was mad. I explained that I just wanted to cook dinner without checking calories or fat or swapping the cream for Quark (fat-free soft cheese).

I wanted to eat like ordinary people eat, and I tried to repair the damage I had done to my children with the many years of damaging diet mentality that I had inflicted on them for most of their lives. Of course, I know what you're thinking,

"You can't lose weight
without going on a diet?"
"Or can you?"

At that point, I honestly did not think you could.

The following week, I went to work where an Indian man would change my thinking forever. This pivotal moment directed me into hours upon hours of research in the form of books, print and audio, podcasts, YouTube videos, blogs, Facebook pages—you name it—I listened to it, read it, and watched it. The things I discovered turned my world upside down.

Six months later, three stone lighter and no dieting, food had become a pleasure again. I felt truly liberated and wanted to shout it from the rooftops. I had so many lightbulb moments along the way. I knew I was not alone on this diet journey, which re-ignited my passion for helping people lose weight.

"One size does not fit all".

Keep reading to find out how you can do the same. I know that along the way, your lightbulb moments will hit you, and they are all so different for all of us. Are you ready to start your study of one.

2

About the course

After discovering so many amazing new things about how my body worked, I decided to jump in and see if these techniques worked! I had read a fantastic theory in a book by ***Dr Bert Herring*** called ***"The Study of 1"*** This effectively meant I was studying myself and what worked personally for me. Working on me was great, but I thought it would be a much better scientific study if others joined me in their studies of 1.

A handful of friends and family all jumped in with me, and we hit the ground running; this trial enabled me to work out that what worked for one might not work for another, so we had to tweak things on our journeys. This was an enormous lightbulb; every plan I had followed was designed to be the same for everyone!

I know I have said it before, but I will repeat it in shouty capitals: -

*"ONE SIZE DOES NOT FIT ALL,
WE ARE ALL DIFFERENT"*

In October 2019, I went to Cyprus for a week with Pete, sat on a sunbed, and wrote a 12-week course to incorporate a plan that suited everyone, as everyone would have lightbulb moments along the way. Every week, they would learn something new and unique about their clever bodies and why it does what it does.

On my return from Cyprus, I launched the course; a lovely lady called Sara allowed me to use her function room in her pub, and we were ready to go; one course turned into four classes, and before I knew it, over 60 people had trusted me on the Learn2Lose journey. The course developed into a day workshop, which I ran from home; this enabled me to get up close and personal with people for a whole day.

I am passionate about spreading this word and bringing the course and all my findings to you in this book. I am writing this in a small farmhouse in northern France; this place holds special memories of my dad, so I couldn't think of a better place to write it.

Grab a pen and paper. It's going to get interactive along the way. To get the best results, you must make notes on your study of 1.

3

Sharing Stories

Q. What do you believe has caused you to be overweight?

Q. What diet plans have you tried in the past?

Q. What effect is being overweight having on your health?

___

___

___

___

Q. What do you believe are the solutions to losing weight?

___

___

___

___

Please consider these questions carefully and write down your answers. I don't mind if you scribble in my book; it will help you start thinking.

Imagine for a minute that you had a leaking pipe in your house, and water was pouring through your ceiling. Would the solution be to go to B and Q and buy some buckets?

No? Why Not? What would you do first?

The first solution would be to find the stop cock and turn the water off, do you agree?

How many reasons did you write down that caused you to be overweight?

Now look at how many solutions you can think of to help you lose weight; these two lists are generally very different:

Here is a list of the common ones. However, your list will be individual for you.

Emotional Eater	*Junk Food*
Portion Sizes	*Depression*
Medication	*Boredom*
Health problems	*Social/Peer pressure*

On the flip side, I find most people answer the solution questions with just two things: -

Eat Less and Move More!

Although this is often written in many ways, it generally comes down to the same thing when we break it down.

If we only fix 1 or 2 leaks but our list of reasons contains 5, 6, 7, or more leaks, what will happen when we turn the water back on? We will still have many leaks to fix, and the problem will not disappear.

I love this analogy as it's a great way to learn how many different leaks we have in our study of 1; remember, this is individual for you, so take some time with your answers so you know what lightbulbs to look for as we go through each section.

4

Current Health Conditions

List any current Health Conditions you are suffering from and any medications you are taking for them.

When you have time, research these conditions and medications to determine what they do and how they work. The reason I ask you to do this is, in my experience, people take medication but often never read the leaflet that tells us how it works; you may discover that this is a big leak for you and an area that we may have to work on in your study of 1.

You must never stop taking a prescribed medication without advice from your GP, but you must always know what it does and why; this goes for all common over-the-counter painkillers as well; you will be amazed at the list of side effects of the humble ibuprofen!

Your Statistics

You can take some time to do this now or later; if you feel comfortable measuring at this point, take some time to dig out a tape measure and write it down. Many people wished they had done this initially but couldn't face it. If now is not the right time and it causes you too much pain, come back to it when the time is right for you. The places to measure are: -

Boobs (yes men you too)
Chest (under boobs for us women)
Waist (an inch above your belly button)
Hips (the biggest bit around your bum)
Arms (the biggest part)
Thigh (the biggest part)

As your study of 1 continues, body re-composition is a real thing. I was freaked out when some of my measurements went up in places, but my clothes were getting looser. I didn't think that could even happen, but it can; when your body starts working right, it tends to put things back where they belong! My boobs have even got more prominent, but my back fat has gone down 5 inches. Work that one out in Bra sizes.

Getting up-to-date health stats from your GP if you haven't had any tests done for a while is also a good idea. The common ones are:

Others may be relevant to your current health conditions; adding them to the list will give you some indicators to work from.

Blood pressure
Cholesterol (a breakdown of LDL & HDL)
HBa1C = blood glucose marker
Thyroid function
Inflammatory markers
Liver function
Kidney function
Full blood count (iron levels)

Photo Profile: this may feel scary right now, and you don't have to look at them if you don't want to!

Photos are, without a doubt, the best way to see visual results that sometimes cannot be quantified on the scales or the tape measure.

When we look in the mirror, we are often so critical of ourselves that it's hard to see what others see.

Pick a set of clothes you wear often and are comfortable in; we can re-create the same photos when you need a visual boost. My recommendations are: -

Front Profile of Face only and Full Body
Side Profile of Face only and Full Body
Rear Profile of Full Body

This was the best thing I have done in my study of 1; I had never been brave enough to do this before. I found a pair of Levi Jeans that Pete bought me during one of my smaller phases (literally no stretch). I used these as a visual; I had to peel them on and off for the photos, and they didn't pull right up; the zip was about 4 inches apart, and now I can wear them out in a public place without losing circulation!

And finally, the Dreaded Scales!

"To Weigh? or not to Weigh? That is the question"

This is a big decision; so many of us have been ruled by the numbers on the scales for the most significant parts of our lives. They do not give a true reflection of our body composition, and they can be very mentally damaging. That said, the choice is yours, but I do have one stipulation: you either weigh every day in the morning after your first pee and record it every day, or you don't weigh at all.

I can detect you thinking that's just weird. This excellent top tip came from Gin Stephens, an inspiring American lady who wrote the book Delay, Don't Deny, and Feast without Fear (I will give a massive shout-out to Gin in my bibliography). Gin taught me to work out my weekly average; I did become a little American at this point and turned my weight into pounds as it's easier to work out.

I suggest looking at the weekly average because of the many fluctuations our weight has daily; our weight fluctuates massively every week; our weight fluctuates by what we have eaten or drunk, and some foods just take on more water to process than others. Looking at the weekly average tells a very different story. I will show you an example of one of my weeks and how you work it out: -

You can see that if my weigh day was weekly on a Wednesday (which it was), I would have potentially thrown the scales out of the bathroom window, hoping to hit everything and everyone in their path!

Monday = 195 Tuesday = 197

Wednesday = 198 Thursday = 195

Friday = 194 Saturday = 195

Sunday = 194

But if you add them all up, it adds up to 1368 pounds, and I then divide that by 7, giving me a weekly average of 195.4. My weekly average the week before was 196.7, so I deducted one from the other, giving me a weight loss this week of -1.3lb; remember, if your moving average is moving even by as little as -0.02, it's still moving. That is not a plateau.

This may seem like hard work, but in true 21st-century style, there's an app for it. I use an app called Happy Scale, but unfortunately, at the time of writing, it was only available on Apple; there is an Android equivalent called My Weight.

If the scales upset you, and you are likely to quit if they don't move, then my top tip is to chuck them in the bin and go by the other methods that are far more effective.

5

What happens in the body when we eat and drink?

So, let's take a closer look. To survive, we must eat and drink, as that is how our body gets energy and stays hydrated, right? But what happens to that food?

> *"Have you ever stopped to consider how your body processes food after it goes into your mouth?"*

Different types of food play very different roles in the body. The best analogy to describe this is by looking at a basic cake recipe.

A basic cake contains what we call the 3 Macro Nutrient Food Groups "***(bear in mind I can't make a cake, so it is very basic!).***"

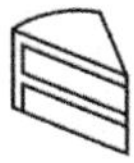

Carbohydrates = Flour and Sugar

Protein = Eggs

Fat = Butter (not margarine, yuk!)

Q. Which one of these is most likely to make us put on weight?

Most of us go for Fat as an answer to this question, as that is what we have been conditioned to think over the years; this is mainly because we use the word Fat to describe ourselves or others around us; it's a descriptive term we have used for many years to describe our physical appearance. This is very far from the truth; the actual answer is the Carbohydrates, the Flour, and the Sugar.

The answer lies in how our body processes these food types very differently and their roles in keeping us functioning daily. That is all it wants to do and in the most energy-efficient way. The problem is it doesn't know what plans you have for it every day, so it tries to second guess our every move before we even decide what's for breakfast!

every single day? the most important role of our body is to keep us alive.

Carbohydrates are what we use as our primary energy source daily; when we eat them, they hit the burning pit of acid in our stomach, and they get turned into Glucose; one thing to bear in mind here is that our body doesn't know if it was a punnet of strawberries or a mars bar once its hit that acid pit down there it pretty much, all comes out looking the same, so don't be fooled that swopping mars bars for fruit will naturally help you lose weight! This energy must be turned into a water-soluble substance to be processed around the body. Unfortunately, we are not Snakes; we cannot move a whole mouse up and down without chewing it first! The Glucose makes its way to the Liver, which is like our Brita Water Filter; it ensures nothing in there will cause us harm, and if there is, it filters it out via our Kidneys.

The Liver is such a vital organ that it does something like 6000 jobs daily!

"I've started to look after mine more since I found that out, I give it a little less vodka".

Now, for some science, I promise to keep it simple as it's essential to understand what your body does with these different Macronutrients.

The liver turns glucose into a substance we call Glycogen, which we send around the body and use as energy. This process seems quite simple, but it's very complex. The body cannot use this energy unless it can be transported into our Cells. Our cellular network is the fundamental function of our body, and nothing happens without the cells being involved. We have trillions of them and make new ones continuously every day.

So, the big question: -

"How do we get this energy into our cells? Annoyingly our clever body keeps the cells locked tight with a big padlock!

To unlock the giant padlock on the cells, we need a magic Key. The magic key is a clever metabolic hormone called Insulin.

Insulin

You may have heard of insulin concerning people with diabetes injecting it, but most of us do not realise how vitally important it is to every function of the body; if we didn't have Insulin in our body, we would die within an average of about five days, without it our cellular network would shut itself down as we would be unable to process any energy from our food. We would go into a state known as Ketoacidosis, which is extremely dangerous and life-threatening.

Discovering that our bodies can only store a certain amount of carbohydrates was a giant light bulb moment for me.

The analogy I find easiest to describe this comes from ***Dr. Jason Fung. His work in*** The Obesity Code and The Diabetes Code is life-changing, and I will credit him in the bibliography.

Dr ***Fung*** calls this our internal fridge;

Q. "If you wanted to make a chicken curry for dinner and you had some chicken in the fridge and some chicken in the freezer, which one would you use first?"

When we eat carbohydrate foods, our fridge starts filling up, and when it's full, we have no room left in the refrigerator; the average-sized human body can store no more than about 2000 calories worth of carbs at any point. When our fridge at home is full, we use our freezer; our body does the same thing with these foods, and insulin helps it on its merry way.

The glycogen that spills out of the fridge gets sent back to the liver and stored as fat first. It then makes its way to the pancreas and fills that with fat, and then it continues to inflame our fat cells one by one as dangerous visceral fat.

This fat is the hard-to-reach stuff we find accumulating, and we never seem to be able to shift, no matter how much weight we lose!

The biggest problem is that we rarely, if ever, get to the point that we empty this fridge, so every time we eat some more carbohydrates, we keep overfilling that fridge and putting more in the fat freezer for a rainy day.

I am guessing you said the chicken in the Fridge, and yes, that is exactly what our body does, too! It likes having plenty of reserves in the freezer for a rainy day, so it doesn't mind you doing that. It likes it as it doesn't have to work very hard.

Our 21st-century diet based on 85% carbs is the biggest issue we now face. We are desperately trying to get in our five a day, looking for low-fat everything and snacking on the so-called health foods like brown rice and whole grain bread, yes carbs, carbs, carbs, even the fruit and veg.

I am not saying we must give them up, but we must examine their role extensively; we will return to them later.

Protein is a bit less complex to explain, but having a moderate amount of it in our daily diet is vitally important. The easiest way to explain protein is to think about a brick wall around your house; if someone smashed into your brick wall, would you choose to mend it with wood? Probably not, as it would look stupid and wouldn't be as strong as it would alter its structure.

Our muscles and organs are the brick walls of our body, and we make them work very hard every day to keep us alive. We must do some continuous maintenance to repair and replenish them, to keep them as fit and healthy as possible; this is protein's job.

Protein gets broken down into what we call Amino acids. I like to think of Amino acids as different-coloured building bricks; we have eight different-coloured bricks.

If we knocked down our red brick wall, we would want a builder to mend it with red brick, yes? If we tried to use a yellow London brick, it would look a bit silly; this is one of the reasons people supplement animal-based products when they become vegetarian or vegan or cut out certain food groups. Unfortunately, not all the eight colours of building bricks are found in all food containing protein, so we need a wide variety to ensure we have all the different building blocks we need when our body needs them.

In basic terms, if your liver is damaged, the best match to repair your liver would be to eat liver.

One thing I have found in my study of 1 is that your body is very good at sending you weird signals when you are deficient in a particular food type. You need to learn to look for the signs; this is like food cravings for bizarre stuff like coal or chalk in a pregnant woman. Craving a packet of crisps can signal salt deficiency, etc.

A couple of bizarre ones for me were the odd desire to eat Brussels sprouts and Liver, which I have never eaten in my 47 years of drawing breath and never thought I would. How's that for strange?

Okay, so that leaves Fat, the one food group we have spent the last 40-odd years being told we should avoid as we were told, ***"Fat makes us fat?"*** Well, I've got big news! Guess what?

"Fat Does NOT Make Us Fat!"

We've been lied to for so long that it's almost criminal. A nasty old scientist named Dr. Ancel Keys devoted his life to convincing the world that Saturated Fat would send us to an early grave!

Suppose you want to do some research here. In that case, you can look deeper into his work on the Heart Health Hypothesis and the Seven Countries study. To summarise, his work has been pulled apart repeatedly, and it has been scientifically proven that Fat is not our enemy. It plays a vital role in our body every day, so our liver must make cholesterol for us if we decide not to eat any.

The work of ***Nina Teicholz*** in her award-winning book ***The Big Fat Surprise*** has opened my eyes to just how much we have had the wool pulled over our eyes.

So, what does Fat do in the body? It plays a few roles. We have a layer of squishy fat just under our skin to keep us warm. That is our subcutaneous fat, or subcut fat for short, and that nasty visceral fat that likes to build up everywhere we don't want it to.

Our liver is so clever that it can turn stored fat into glucose to feed our brains. If we have no glycogen stores, this process is known as Gluconeogenesis. We can also use fat as a primary energy source again with the help of the liver, producing something called Ketone bodies, so our bodies go into fat-burning mode known as Ketosis.

Without Fat, we would die; this is why the liver can make cholesterol, again, because it just won't take the chance of relying on you eating it for it to be able to keep you alive.

Cast your mind back a few chapters when we talked about the cellular network, the fundamental function of our body, and the engine room to every single function we perform every day.

The trillions of cells in the body need to be strong and healthy to carry stuff around our bloodstream and perform all those functions we need to keep us alive; our cells work hard like little trojans every second of every day. To make the cell membranes strong and healthy, we must have good quality fat, aka our good cholesterol; if our cells were water soluble, it would be a disaster as our blood is also water-soluble; this would be like using a chocolate teapot on a hot day., so we need fat to make our cells. There is a bit more science there, but that's the way I find it easiest to remember how vital fat is.

When we have damaged cells or cells that don't form properly, this puts us at risk of many common cellular degenerative diseases and increases our risks of tumours growing from unused, damaged cells.

Recent research has shown that many of the common cognitive diseases, such as dementia, Alzheimer's, and Parkinson's disease, are caused by poor cell formation.

Therefore, we cannot live on rabbits alone. Rabbits are herbivores and do not have any fat, so we would die if we tried to live on a diet of rabbits alone!

It's time to get your pen and paper back out or scribble on the book.

Previous Diets

Q. What was your most successful previous diet?

Q. How much weight did you lose roughly?

Q. How much weight did you regain?

Q. What made you give it up?

You may be thinking this a bit cruel, especially the weight regain question; when I was at my lowest, I had started to believe it was me. I couldn't lose weight anymore, I always blamed myself, and the internal dialogue would start telling me I was useless, I'm greedy, I've got no will-power, bla bla bla, you know how that little story in our head goes! And that is, without people around us giving us their two pennies worth, we do not need anyone else telling us how rubbish we are at diets! We tell ourselves that enough. Thank you very much!

So, the interesting point about this is that we have all succeeded in losing weight on various diets at some point in our lives. I shared my story of my attempts at the beginning of the book. The big key here for me was: -

We are not stupid!

We are an intelligent nation; if someone said to follow this plan, and I guarantee you will lose weight and look like Elle McPherson, a Victoria's Secret model, or some drop-dead gorgeous Instagram influencer, I'm sure a fair proportion of us would do it. I know I would have done it.

So, we know we can follow a plan as we all have; we know we can lose weight as we all have, but why do we give it up? Because they are too hard to follow long term? That is the main reason I have come up with over the last 20 years of listening to people's reasons for not getting results; the big thing I have found so strange is why we blame ourselves and not the diet inventors for making their stupid diets so hard to follow!

In conclusion, a massive light bulb moment for me here was that I could only do something I could do for life; otherwise, this would end up in the long list of failed attempts to lose three stone, which was now 4.5 stone instead of 3! Eek. I couldn't do another diet; I knew my naughty schoolgirl mindset would creep in every time I went on holiday or Christmas or I broke a fingernail!

6

Eat Less and move more

This is still, without doubt, the most common advice given to people who want to lose weight; I, too, believed that it was a simple law that if you burned off more than you put in the law of thermodynamics, it had to mean that you lost weight, yes? Sadly no!

Q. What is a Calorie and how is it determined?

This theory is built around energy consumption and expenditure and the calories in versus calories out model that we have all tried so many times, and it just didn't work long term.

A calorie is a unit of Energy determined by the rate at which it burns. Working out how many calories something is is more like a science experiment than something we could do at home! They place food in a tube, set fire to it, and record how hot and how long it burns to simulate what would happen in the body when we ate that same food.

It was never designed to help people lose weight; it was a system devised to calculate the energy in food rather than whether it would make us gain or lose weight.

The human body does not set fire to our food when we digest it. So, this process gives us an indication of why this model is so flawed.

So why doesn't it work?

Q. Would we lose the same weight if I followed a 1000 kcal per day Kit Kat diet and my daughter Daisy followed a 1000 kcal per day Celery Diet?

According to the law of thermodynamics, 1000 kcal is 1000 kcal regardless of where it came from, but if we go back to the model where we broke down the macronutrients in the cake, we can see that the body treats foods very differently.

The best way to explain this is to imagine you have a scorching cup of tea; I'm sure you have all dunked a biscuit and dropped it in your tea at some stage. I know I have! When you get to the bottom of that cup of tea, there is very little evidence of the biscuit left; it dissolves into the hot tea very quickly; this simulates what would happen in the stomach to our Kit Kat. Remember, it's a burning pit of acid in our stomach around pH. 1.5 that's fiery.

Now take the celery, for the love of god, that stringy stuff never breaks down. It's what we call insoluble fibre, which we will talk more about later; the body knows that when something doesn't break down in the burning pit of acid, it can't get through the Brita water filter in our liver to be processed into energy, this is where the body is clever it sends it out via the small intestine and to the bowel so we don't absorb those calories in the body as we do with the Kit Kat.

Even if you took the same piece of celery and ate it in two different ways, the body would absorb the calories very differently; if we ate the first piece of celery raw, we would chew it a lot to wind it down, and if we took another piece and turned it into a soup and blended it, the body would have to do far less work to process it so that it would expend less energy. Unfortunately, none of this is considered in the basic rules of Calories in, Calories out.

Alcohol

Alcohol plays an entirely different role here; if we take pure alcohol like spirits, i.e., vodka, gin, whiskey, etc., it has no nutritional profile, so no carbohydrates, no protein, and no fat, so it has no macronutrients that the body uses for its various jobs, this makes it what we call an Empty Calorie, this is effectively a calorie that doesn't have any jobs to do in the body. It still contains calories, so it is still an energy source. The body cannot ignore these calories as they have been consumed, so it has to do something with them; it ponders for a while. It has to go through the Brita water filter in the liver as it's picked up as a toxin; it then works out that it's not carbs, protein, or fat. This takes a bit more time to work out, and then it realises that it cannot store these calories, so it puts them first in the queue to be used as a quick energy source. This always poses the question, why do we rarely see an overweight alcoholic? The answer is they don't generally eat! Eating's cheating!

So, in a scenario where we would find ourselves having a few cheeky vinos each night with dinner, the body would store the dinner as that's easy for it to do while it uses up the empty calories first for energy. This is why we often find we gain weight when we drink alcohol, but it takes longer to show up on the scales as it takes longer to process through the body.

The story's moral is: If you want to go out and drink, don't eat! No, not really. I'm only kidding. If alcohol features heavily in your life, you may need to look at this area, as some of us struggle to metabolise it.

So that's calories in. What about calories out? That's a whole different ball game!

Q. How many calories do you need to burn off through exercise per day to lose 1lb of Fat per week? "500"

Yes, you need to burn 500 calories daily to lose just 1lb per week; to put that into perspective, that is the equivalent of a 5k jog or a 2.5-hour walk every day.

If you went out and did a 5k jog every day, and you came to me and jumped on my scales, and I told you that you had lost just 1lb, I can almost guarantee I would have to duck pretty quick before you attempted to throw those scales at my head and knock me clean out!

So, this is back to that simple theory of thermo dynamics again: if we expend more than we consume, we should, in theory, lose weight at a rate of around 1lb per every 3500 calories burned.

This is a straightforward mathematical equation, but our body doesn't work that way; it has some very clever, sneaky tricks that mess up this simple mathematical equation.

Remember we talked about how the body's basic plan is to keep us alive every day, and it doesn't consider what we want in our heads? This is one of those times where it will always try and second guess you; if the body feels threatened by you trying to burn up too many calories, it will do all manner of things to ensure that doesn't happen.

The first thing it does is ramp up the production of our hunger hormone, Ghrelin; we will talk more about Ghrelin later; this is where the term working up an appetite comes from. It will also make us less likely to expend as much energy for the rest of the day on other functions by ramping up our sleep hormone, Melatonin; this clever trick ensures we get plenty of rest to give us time to repair and replenish damaged muscle tissue and conserve more energy. The other smart trick it can play is lowering our heart rate, which lowers blood pressure. One last one, it can drop our body core temperature; this is why we see marathon runners wrapped in silver foil blankets at the end of a race as we run the risk of going hypothermic if our core body temperature drops below 35 degrees, which will in turn cause the body to start shutting down. Clever stuff, huh?

The body's rule is that if we burn 500 calories, it will do all it can to replenish or conserve 600 calories, which is the best way it knows how. Remember, it wants to keep you alive the best way it knows!

How we metabolise food also changes when we put the body under stress through exercise. Our stress hormone cortisol ramps up when it detects stress (the fight or flight response). This, in turn, raises our blood glucose; when blood glucose rises, we need the hormone insulin to

regulate it, and good old insulin makes us feel stupidly hungry so it can help the body replenish its fat stores, so yes, you've guessed it, keep us alive. It will never rely on you to do the right thing as the body doesn't trust you; it keeps these little clever tricks for times it knows it needs to protect you from yourself.

So, you see, when you pound the streets or the treadmill or shake your booty in a Zumba class, you may think you are expending a certain amount of energy based on the basic rules of thermodynamics. Still, your body has completely different ideas; our biggest problem is working out what it will do and when!

So, when you exercise forget how many Kcals you are burning, and always do something you love with people you love while you are laughing.

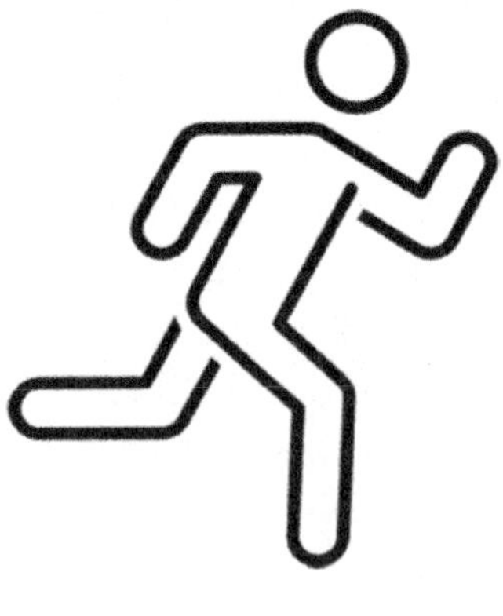

7

The Metabolism

Q. What is the Metabolism? Can we touch it? Can we feel it? Does it start? Does it stop?

I get many different answers when I ask this question in a group. We hear about this continuously in the 21st century, but we are still waiting for someone to tell us what it is!

The direct translation of the Metabolism is: -

"State of Change"

It cannot stop. Otherwise, we would be dead; we can't touch it or see it, it is not one thing: it's a combination of many things.

The best way I have found to describe it is as follows: -

It is a makeup of around 40 different hormones that respond to changes in our body; these are known as

Metabolic Responses, i.e. if we eat cake, our glucose levels rise, so our Metabolic Response to increasing blood glucose is the excretion of the metabolic hormone Insulin to regulate it. When a mother gives birth to a baby, the metabolic response is to excrete a hormone called Oxytocin, our love hormone; the baby also excretes Oxytocin when it's near its mother. This is one of the reasons a mother can settle her crying baby easier than anyone else. When we exercise, we excrete Serotonin, known as the feel-good hormone. It affects mood. This is why people get hooked on exercise, as they love the feel-good feeling it gives them.

These Metabolic responses happen all day, every day, in our bodies, and our actions are very much responsible for triggering them.

Some of the everyday things people say are: -

"I can't lose weight because I have a slow metabolism" or "you have to eat breakfast to kick start your metabolism",

or the most common diet myth,

"If you don't eat you will ruin your metabolism!"

These statements are all myths and misconceptions, and they have paved the way for mass manufacturers and big pharma to trick us into paying for products and services to speed up our metabolisms! These products are a big waste of money! A great book is Lies My Doctor Told Me by Dr. Ken Berry. This book will help you understand how we have been tricked for many years.

What we do need to do, though, is help our metabolisms work as effectively as possible; we know that when our metabolic responses are not working correctly, we massively struggle with many things, and losing weight is a big one.

Resting Metabolic / Basal Rate

Q. What is our Resting/ Basal Metabolic Rate?

Resting Metabolic Rate, or Basal Metabolic Rate as often termed, plays an important role here.

This is effectively the amount of Energy (calories) our body needs to do its essential daily functions: eat, sleep, breathe, keep our heart beating and our brain functioning, and all the other bits in between.

Q. Can you work out your RMR/ BMR in actual calories?

You may be surprised to know that our Brains require the most energy, needing around 300 calories daily to keep us alive!

Yes, you can. You will find there are many different expensive sets of scales and gadgets on the market that claim to do this for you, but in truth, to work it out accurately, you need some technical, expensive machinery; the most accurate form of testing is known as a ***Direct Calorimetry Test,*** this involves sitting in an airtight chamber for around an hour with minimal movement which allows the machine to analyse how much body heat and carbon dioxide is expended. An actual resting metabolic rate can be determined from these measurements. That's all very expensive and not widely available for the average you and me, so most of us use the essential functions that are relatively easy to work out using an app or some funky bathroom scales.

Q. What things determine our Basic Resting/Basal Metabolic Rate?

These four variables are used to calculate the essential energy expenditure of a person at rest, i.e., when they are not doing anything physical but staying alive.

1. Age
2. Gender
3. Weight
4. Height

Age 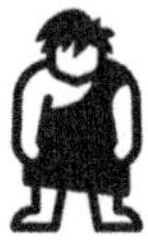

Age plays a role as it changes how much energy we burn at rest. Due to the ageing process, our muscle mass starts to degenerate at a rate of around 1% per year from the age of about 35. We can prolong this by staying as fit and healthy as possible, but we cannot defy ageing. When muscle mass degenerates, muscle turns to Fat, and Fat doesn't need as much energy to keep it stable as lean muscle tissue. Therefore, people start to eat much less as they age; they do not need as much energy to stay alive.

Gender

Gender is probably the most interesting one I've found, and it surprises people. The government guidelines for calories for men and women are 2000 for women and 2500 for men, but nobody ever takes any notice, and we don't stop questioning why men get to eat more without putting on weight!

Things concerning equality and evolution have changed over the centuries. We now have a 5ft intestine as we learned to cook, and we suffer from impacted wisdom teeth as we don't have to chew raw foods 50-odd times a bite, but the long and short of it is our bodies were made for very different reasons, and this has not changed. Women were made to reproduce and, in turn, given boobs and childbearing hips to store more body fat; this is to protect the unborn child and us during the gestation period. As we discovered, with age, the fat-to-muscle ratio in our body determines how much energy we need to keep us alive. A woman's average body fat percentage is around 29-36%, and a lean man's average body fat percentage is approximately 8-18%. This means that a woman should eat, on average, a third less at each meal to remain the same weight as a man.

If you think about this logically, it's not taught in schools. If you raise two children, a boy and a girl, when they hit puberty, they should adjust what they eat accordingly so either one doesn't lose weight or gain weight depending on what gender they are; this is often apparent when you hear stories of families saying my son is tall and skinny and eats like a horse, but my daughter struggles with her weight.

The biggest issue in modern society is how often we eat out or order takeout. I am sure you have never seen a separate male and female menu in a restaurant or takeaway, and most servings are man-size portions; human nature tells us it is polite to eat what's on our plates, and if we are paying good money for it, we certainly do not want to waste it!

This is often seen after a holiday as you tend to find women always gain more weight than men on holiday since we eat out in restaurants or go all-inclusive and don't want to waste our money. We find we spend most of the holiday eating man-size portions!

Weight

Weight is one of the big reasons we Yoyo diet. Think of this basic scenario: if I weighed 20 stones and ran up a big hill, or if I weighed ten stones and ran up the same hill, which would take more energy? The 20-stone version of me or the 10-stone version of me.

> ***"As we lose weight our body will want and need less food".***

Yes, the 20-stone version of me needs more energy to run up the hill due to the weight it needs to carry. The big area that gets gravely overlooked here is that our body requires less energy to keep us alive when we lose weight.

So, in the weight loss scenario, this becomes a real problem. We start a diet, and we get used to losing weight at a steady rate, but as our weight starts to decrease, we now have to start reducing the food going in or increasing the energy we expend through exercise; the problem is that we already know from our calories in calories out discussion this isn't that easy as our body has different ideas, this is why over the long term calorie restriction diets do not lead to sustainable weight loss. The best example of this can be found in the ***Women's Health Initiative study in 2006***, which was the largest of its type ever carried out in the US. They took over 45,000 women to try and determine specific health outcomes based on weight loss and different kinds of diet; it lasted eight years and was a controlled study costing the US taxpayer 700 million USD; in the three groups they studied, a calorie restriction diet, a low-fat diet and an exercise based diet they had to report back what they were eating and were followed up with regular counselling sessions and support along the way, The results were supposed to find the perfect diet to recommend to the American women to prevent Coronary Heart Disease, reduce Hypertension and blood cholesterol levels and maintain a healthy Body Mass index.

The outcomes were quite shocking. Initially, there was some weight loss, but over the extended period, the average weight loss was just ¼ pounds over the eight years. More shocking still, there were no positive health outcomes, and some groups raised overall mortality in other areas, such as cancer and other lifestyle diseases.

The other study that highlights these findings is the ***Greatest Loser Study***. This one is well worth a read; this famous TV show produced a documentary six years later highlighting that the people who had lost massive amounts of weight on the show had pretty much gained most if not all, their weight back and some had gained even more weight. I know what you think: they went back to eating junk and not exercising; well, in fact, no, they continued to follow the plan and even upped the exercise and reduced the calorie intake even further, but that clever body plays tricks and can shut down certain functions decreasing the resting metabolic rate to protect us, on average the metabolic rates of the contestants had decreased by up to 800 calories per day and remained reduced for several years after the initial weight loss, even after they gained the weight back. This is the true definition of our body going into starvation mode, not skipping breakfast as we have been led to believe for so many years.

Height

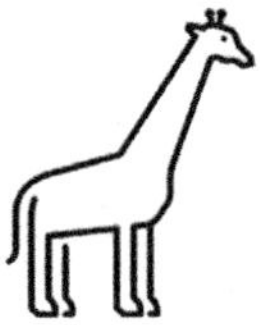

Height is simple; imagine this scenario: we have a 6-foot-tall woman and a 4-foot-tall woman. Which one is going to need more energy to stay alive?

Yes, the 6-foot-tall woman will need more energy (calories) because her blood has to travel much further around her body to get where it needs to go.

We all know someone extremely tall who can eat like a horse and never gains any weight! I have large carving knives that are particularly effective for these people! I am only kidding; please don't attack the tall, skinny ones. They aren't necessarily healthy, just thin!

So, in conclusion, this was a lot to process, and I've found many people have big lightbulb moments here; if you're getting older, female overweight, and didn't get given the tall gene at birth, your resting metabolic rate will be much lower. It may help you to understand why you find it hard to lose weight with calorie-restrictive diets.

Other factors can affect how our Metabolic Responses work in our Body; please tick which ones apply to you; this will help you build up a bigger picture of how many leaks you may have in your pipework that we need to fix: -

Calorie restrictive dieting
Excessive exercise/training
Extreme or rapid weight loss
Insulin resistance
Hormone imbalances i.e., thyroid function
Stress / Anxiety / Depression
Pre-existing medical condition
Taking medication

The more ticks you have, the more leaks we must fix.

This knowledge will allow us to move forward and work on each area to get our metabolic responses working correctly.

"Knowledge is power but
only if you use it",

8

Appetite correction / Body set weight

This was another massive lightbulb-lighting moment for me, and you should do some further reading here. Dr Bert Herring has a fantastic book called The Power of AC. He writes in straightforward terms and explains many different theories on this subject.

I will keep this simple without the technical science stuff. We have to remember that we are clever individuals and all our body parts are linked to other body parts; this is no different when it comes to our appetite; we eat because our brain sends a signal to the stomach to produce a hormone that physically creates a feeling of hunger, this process is so we do not starve ourselves to death, we also have another hormone that sends a signal to the brain from the stomach to tell us to stop eating when we are full up or satiated. These two hormones are known as Ghrelin and

Leptin. We will look at them again later in more depth. These essential functions are given to us as in-built survival mechanisms, one so we don't starve ourselves to death and the other so we do not eat until we explode, as in the case of the ***Monty Python Sketch Mr Creosote*** my dad's favourite saying, when he felt like he couldn't eat one more thing.

"Just one more wafer-thin mint"

These mechanisms are controlled by a part of the brain known as the Hypothalamus. This is like the thermostat in our head that sorts out what, when, where, and why we eat a bit.

This clever system is impressive when it works correctly, helping us regulate portion sizes, cravings, and weight.

This is another area where the body can play clever little tricks with those Metabolic Responses. As we discussed earlier, working up an appetite alerts the thermostat that we are using a bit more energy than we need to, so its response is to ramp up the hunger signals to make us put a bit more back in. We probably wouldn't notice this happening, but it can dramatically affect our weight.

The biggest issue I've found in this area is that when we have endured so many different calorie-restrictive diets and tried so hard to burn off those pesky calories exercising, more times than we care to shake a stick at, our Metabolic Responses can be a bit shall we say: -

"Confused".

Our modern-day society has taught us to eat for many different reasons besides hunger, mainly because the clock says 8,12, and 6, or anywhere between.

When we ignore these hormones over time by eating when we are not hungry and not stopping when we are satisfied, they get fed up and stop working correctly. This is a term known as Metabolic Syndrome, and it affects all of us who have or are struggling to lose weight.

Body set weight

Body set weight is the other tricky little metabolic stunt our body plays on us; I was almost angry with my body when I learnt about this. Our body likes to remain in what is called,

Homeostasis

Homeostasis is effectively a fancy name for everything staying the same. The body likes everything to stay the same, so it doesn't have to work hard. The body can perform the primary function of keeping us alive every day with minimal effort.

The problem here is that the body knows that to protect you, you must always think of that rainy day when you might get poorly and not be able to eat, or we might have another world war. Rationing gets put back in place, there's a significant famine, or the food shops close for a whole day! And we might starve. Most of us live in an abundant society and have enough food in our cupboards to survive for a long time, but our bodies don't always recognise this. The average human body with no weight to lose has around -

100,000 calories in stored fat at any one point,

This would last you around 60 days without you eating a single thing! So, when we talked about burning off 3500 calories per week to lose 1lb of body fat, it felt a bit put out as it worked very hard to get them into storage for you in the first place!

For every pound of excess fat, you can multiply it by an average of 3500 calories per pound, so the average human with 20 pounds to lose would have around 170,000 calories worth of energy stored on their body; this would last them about 100 days without physically needing any food and without harming their health.

This is where the body's set weight kicks in; when our body starts to feel the effects of weight loss and fat storage depletion happening, it doesn't like it; it feels immediately under threat; this is why rapid or extreme weight loss creates such desperate measures as in ***the greatest loser study.*** The body will always try replenishing those fat stores by ramping up hunger and reducing our metabolic rate. This is to get us back to our body-set weight or homeostasis. Often, this is the weight we have been at the most in our lives; most of us find that when we suffer weight regain, it's usually a few pounds more than we lost in the first place! This is another second-guess trick by the body, just in case you try that cunning stunt again! This will push the body set weight up over time and make it even harder to lose weight the next time we try. ***The Minnesota starvation study*** is an excellent example of this theory and shows how clever the human body is at protecting us when it feels under threat.

This is an excellent self-regulatory mechanism. If everything is working right, it tends to keep skinny people skinny and overweight people overweight! It's rubbish if your genetics put you in the overweight group!

This theory has been proven repeatedly with animals and various twin studies. ***Gary Taubes*** talks about the different species of animals in his book ***Why We Get Fat And What To Do About It.*** Animals in the wild have the same ecosystem as us, but the ones that are meant to be fat remain fat without storing excess visceral fat, like an elephant, and the fat ones that need vast amounts of excess stored fat, like Blue whales, do this efficiently. A Lion living in the wild will only leave its spot lazing in the sunshine when it really must eat to survive, and it will never overeat; otherwise, it would gain weight, and something would eat it! Certain species of animals must store body fat to survive. Hibernation and research have shown that when these animals, such as squirrels, are put on a calorie-restrictive diet during the pre-hibernation period, they still gain the fat they need to survive as they are genetically preprogrammed to sacrifice energy in other areas. Fat storage takes priority, so they stay as a species. Some shocking laboratory tests have been done on hibernating animals that have been starved to death, and they often die with lots of stored body fat as their body knows that is what they must do to survive.

In conclusion, Humans are the only Mammals that have learned how to mess up this self-regulatory system, and the outcome has been chronic disease and a worldwide obesity epidemic.

Q. What do you think may have had a big impact on this in the last 35 years?

The most significant contributing factor has been our shift in our Macro nutrient food groups; around 85% of our modern diet now comes from Carbohydrates! This is mainly due to mass manufacture, food science, and the billion-pound diet industry messing with our heads daily! We will talk more about that later.

9

Hormones aka gremlins

So often, Hormones get blamed for many things going wrong in our bodies; when we go to the GP, they offer very little help in this area, and getting a referral to an endocrine specialist is like getting blood from a stone! Well, in a nutshell, yes, our hormones or metabolic responses, to give them the correct term, impact every function our body performs.

The following page lists some of our metabolic responses' most significant effects on our health.

This is not an exhaustive list; there are many more, and I am sure you can think of some to add to it.

Mood	*Fatigue*
Sleep	*Hunger*
Immune system	*Muscle strength*

Stress / Anxiety	Body temperature
Fat burning/storing	Blood glucose
Hair growth or loss	Weight loss or gain
Neuron transmission	Acne
Reproduction	

Four big ones are associated mainly with their effects on our weight and how we feel: -

Thyroid

The thyroid hormones T3, T4, and TSH are vital for regulating fat; if these hormones are not responding correctly, it's generally termed as overactive or underactive; it can have a massive impact on weight loss, weight gain, chronic fatigue, and even hair loss, often you hear people saying I wish I had the one that makes you lose weight not the one that makes it hard to lose weight, trust me you wouldn't, it's a severe condition and has some horrible side effects.

The sex hormones

The sex hormones testosterone, estrogen, and progesterone are linked to all sorts of weird and wonderful functions. If they are low or high, they can affect mood, hair loss or growth, weight loss or gain, sleep, reproduction, low libido, fibroids, anxiety, depression, acne, thyroid dysfunction, hot flushes, headaches, migraines, endometriosis. I'm sure I've missed some; you get the picture, in any case. They play a vital role. The big thing with this little gang of hormones is that they like to chop and change through different times of our lives, and sometimes we have no choice; our age has one of the most considerable effects here as these hormones go through cycles starting with puberty through to menopause. From the age of 35, our sex hormones begin to decline, but this can happen much earlier or later, and it can have a very negative effect on our physical and mental well-being.

Certain health conditions can have a massive impact, such as the removal of the ovaries, a complete hysterectomy, and specific prostate cancer treatments in men. These can dramatically affect our production of these hormones, and alternative therapies are required to regulate them to avoid adverse health effects artificially.

Trials on removing the ovaries of mice have proven that a lack of estrogen changes how the body metabolises fat. This causes the mice to store body fat and gain weight even on a calorie-restrictive diet. The mice also became far more sedentary; scientists believe this was to preserve energy due to the changes in metabolic hormones. This is thought to be one of the reasons weight gain is often more prolific during menopause or after the removal of the female reproductive system.

Cortisol

Cortisol is a big one. Otherwise known as the stress hormone, it was given to us as a survival mechanism to protect us from harm. When the body senses a threat, it triggers a response known as the -

fight or flight response!

If you think back to hunter-gatherer times, this survival mechanism sprang into action, so you had the energy to stand and fight for your dinner or know when you are on the losing team and be away on your toes and run. Hence the term fight or flight!

I always liken this to fighting a grizzly bear; we have baby grizzly bears that are cute and fluffy; we might fancy our chances with those, and then we have the Mumma grizzly protecting her young. She's a whole different ball game. When the brain detects a rise in cortisol, a signal is sent to the brain to find some glucose. Our brain also knows that our primary source of energy is glucose. To protect us, it has a funky little trick up its sleeve; it keeps glucose stored in all manner of weird locations in the body, ready for these grizzly bear moments. Some places, it keeps glucose hidden; I can't even pronounce!

At this grizzly bear-facing moment, the metabolic response is to ramp up Cortisol. The fight or flight responder kicks in the body, searches for some glucose and dumps that glucose directly into our bloodstream; if you remember from earlier when our blood glucose rises, our body has another metabolic response as it needs insulin to enter to regulate that elevated glucose level. Insulin makes us feel stupidly, insatiably hungry. This is often why stress makes us want to comfort eat, and we crave sugary carbohydrate-based food; insulin knows these are the quickest foods to replenish the glucose we just used fighting that Mumma grizzly bear.

The biggest issue in today's fast-paced world is that we often face several Mumma grizzlies and a few baby grizzlies daily! Have you been through an airport lately or up and down the motorway? There are a few right there! Don't even get me started on money, kids, health, work, relationships. Our metabolic systems were not designed to cope with the extreme stress we must deal with today! Fact!

High circulating cortisol levels will cause your body to hang on to every bit of stored body fat. That is without mentioning the many other areas of your life and health it likes to play tricks with; it can raise our heart rate, which in turn increases blood pressure, affect your sleep and mood, cause headaches and migraines, affect sex drive, and play havoc with our inflammatory markers.

Insulin

Insulin is the fat hormone. This is, without a shadow of a doubt, the daddy of the metabolic responses; you will hear this hormone rise to fame over the next ten years as more and more research hits the headlines. I know I only ever thought about diabetes and how it is used to control the condition. It is crucial in our body and plays several roles, without insulin our body would start to shut down on a cellular level at breakneck speed, the average human body would be dead within five days without insulin production, and it would effectively start eating itself in a state known as Keto Acidosis.

The biggest issue with insulin is how it overrides many of our other metabolic responses.

If you remember earlier, we talked about our internal fridge and the body's lack of ability to store too much glycogen; this significantly affects our insulin production. When our internal fridge is full, and fat starts backing up around the body, it can cause the insulin to behave peculiarly; the body-responsive way of dealing with a carbohydrate overload is to alert the pancreas that it needs more insulin. I always believed that insulin and glucose came hand in hand! But no, I was wrong in this belief. It is possible to have a high level of circulating insulin coupled with a low blood glucose level.

This is known as Hyperinsulinemia; this condition is rarely diagnosed due to an extreme lack of adequate endocrine testing. I have firsthand experience of the effects of high insulin levels as both my daughters have acute insulin resistance.

High circulating insulin levels often build up when the body's Metabolic Responses are not working correctly. Some of the symptoms of this condition are: -

Weight Gain
Insatiable Hunger
Lack of Concentration (brain fog)
Anxiety / Panic
Fatigue
Lack of Motivation
Metabolic Syndrome

Hyperinsulinemia is the precursor to insulin resistance, a knock-on effect of insulin not doing its job correctly, resulting in a high level of circulating insulin remaining in the bloodstream.

The mad part of this sorry tale of insulin is its role in managing Diabetes, Type 1 and Type 2. Less than 100 years ago, we discovered that we could extract insulin from a pig and inject it into a human to save lives, which is extraordinary if you think about it!

Think back to the beginning and our discussion on our leaking pipe. When someone is diagnosed with type 1 diabetes, they are immediately prescribed insulin and advised to count carbs and adjust their insulin per regular blood glucose testing results. This system creates a constant daily spiral of peaks and troughs in blood glucose, rising after food and blood glucose dipping after insulin is administered. It is tough to manage and comes with lots of health issues if poorly managed. Diabetes type 2 is generally diet-controlled initially, which is often unsuccessful; the next course of treatment is various medications, the main one being metformin, which neutralises the glucose in the gut and makes the body think it needs less insulin. This usually works for a time, and then the final inevitable course of treatment is insulin injections to regulate the raised glucose levels in the blood. The big issue here is that the pre-cursor to insulin resistance, which causes type 2 diabetes, is hyperinsulinemia, and the cause of hyperinsulinemia is producing too much insulin; here's the bit that's hard to get your head around: -

"To manage the condition, we administer more insulin! "

Do you see the problem if our leak was caused by too much insulin circulating in the blood? Administering more insulin to fix the problem is like buying a considerable bucket at the hardware store! We cannot fix the problem of too much insulin with more insulin; in fact, it worsens the situation. Eventually, the glucose becomes resistant to the insulin, and blood glucose remains elevated; the insulin is then raised to regulate the higher circulating glucose, and the vicious cycle begins.

Insulin resistance is the inevitable result of hyperinsulinemia, which is the cause of diabetes type 2, but also the cause of chronic obesity; they are the same conditions. They manifest themselves differently in different people at other times of their lives.

Diabetes type 2 and chronic obesity are both curable dietary conditions, not progressive diseases. We need to learn to improve insulin sensitivity and resolve our broken metabolic responses, and we can cure the obesity crisis!

This was my most significant lightbulb moment with my two daughters. I knew in my heart of hearts that their weight issues were not solely about the food they were eating, but logic was telling me it must be about food. What else could it be? We always find our way back to the laws of thermodynamics and calories in versus calories out; they must have too many calories coming in and not be burning them off!

In Daisy's case, she was working 50 hours a week or more on her feet in a commercial kitchen and mucking out a horse in between, her split shifts, if 10 hours a day on your feet running around a kitchen isn't enough to burn off some calories, what more could we do!

Daisy's level of circulating insulin in her blood had reached epic levels; I later discovered that she could have lived on lettuce every day and still not lost weight! I can distinctly remember her first appointment with the bariatric surgeon at Kings College; she looked at my terrified 18-year-old daughter and said what diets have you tried? Daisy told her she had tried many different things, but the weight came straight back, with a bit more besides! She looked at her and said: -

> ***"Well, it's not hard, is it? You just have to eat less and move more. Why don't you try that?"***

My face must have been a picture! I sat there feeling so sorry for her. The surgeon played the blame game repeatedly, just like all the other medical professionals we had seen. We left her office, and I vowed to prove that lady wrong. That day, I wholeheartedly thought about why our bodies do what they do.

10

Healthy food vs Unhealthy food

When I came back from my holiday back in August 2019, I vowed that I didn't want to buy crap diet food anymore. I was convinced this was not helping me, but there were things I didn't know then. I soon discovered I was right to make this decision; what I uncovered next was probably the most challenging change for me but the one with the quickest result.

Q. What is a pre-chewed food?

Something that is pre-chewed means it didn't start life looking like it does now, so back to the Kit Kats and Celery, the Kit Kats don't grow, we can't pick them, they start life looking very different, and a big factory chews all the bits up for us before they put it back together and put it in a pretty packet and market it to death until we think we cannot live without it!

I read ***Gin Stephens's book Feast without Fear*** and studied the blue zones of the world where people live the longest; they pretty much all have one thing in common: they eat whole food, they eat local food, and they eat seasonally; there is not a pre-chewed food in sight! I thought about the foods in my diet for the past 25 years. Most of my food was some new box of something that was going to aid my weight loss, like chocolate brownies that had more protein and only 90 calories or little packs of pasta I could tip in a cup and pour hot water on if a recipe asked for cream, butter or oil it would be substituted with a low-fat alternative or a 1kcal spray. My most significant substitute was swopping sugar for artificial sweetener in everything: sweetener in my tea, diet coke, low-fat, artificially sweetened yoghurts, skimmed milk, low-fat cheese, you name it I was a mass manufacturer's dream.

The result of eating these foods for the past 25 or more years has made me bigger than I had ever been! So how the hell was I going to give them up and lose weight?

Low-fat foods

Low-Fat Foods***: Remember, earlier in the book,*** I talked about our shift in Macronutrients and a move to a much higher percentage of carbohydrates in our modern-day diet.

When we adopted the low-fat diet in the late '80s and early '90s (I like to call it the ***Rosemary Conley Era***), we all got very clever at reading nutritional labels. We were encouraged to look for saturated fat, added salt, and sugar, and little traffic lights started appearing on the front of packets to convince us if something was good or bad to eat. These theories have been bulldozed into our brains for 40 or more years!

This was walking right into the hands of the mass manufacturers and the ultra-processed nightmare we now live with. Once they realised they could divert our eyes to this little box on the back of the packets, they also quickly learned to manipulate the figures on them to trick us into thinking food was good for us when, in fact, the truth was very different.

For example, let's take a full-fat yoghurt; its texture is thick, creamy, and yummy. We now think fat is the enemy, but we still want to eat yoghurt. Voila, low-fat yoghurt was to take the diet world by storm. Stupidly, we did not stop to ask what they did to it! How did they remove the fat and still make it taste like yoghurt?

Have you ever put your potatoes on to boil for your Sunday roasties, gone away to do something else, and run back in screaming for the Potatoes? If you haven't humour me as I have many times! The result is a saucepan of gloopy water known as potato starch; yes, your low-fat frankin food manufacturers (foods made by Frankenstein) must find some filler, and the cheapest, easiest, most widely available filler is starch and usually from potatoes. This decreases the fat content, so the nutritional label looks impressive, but we never stopped to think about its effect on carbohydrates. Remember what we said earlier: fat is not the enemy; fat doesn't make us fat. Think back to the section where we discussed what carbohydrates do in our body, and hey presto, we have a perfect storm in a teacup! Or yoghurt pot, as the case may be. We took the good stuff out and didn't even consider that what they put back in was doing us more harm. Take a little look at your fridge or cupboard for all the low-fat alternatives you have bought in the hope of losing weight! I promise you; you will be horrified. I know I was.

Artificial sweeteners

Sweeteners ***are*** the most used substitute for sugar and one of the most used artificial foods worldwide. It is almost impossible to find mass-manufactured food and drink that doesn't contain some form of artificial sweetener. The introduction of the sugar tax has exacerbated this beyond belief in recent years.

This was another of my vast lightbulb switching-on moments; you must return to man's creation to better understand.

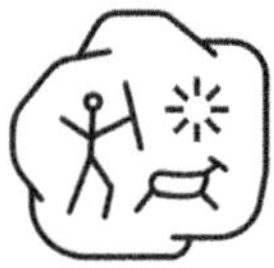

Q. Why were we created with a sense of taste and a sense of smell?

Our senses were given to us, so we didn't poison ourselves; if something tasted very nasty on our tongue, it sent an immediate warning signal to our brain to eject it immediately by spitting it out; this is also why we do not choose to eat dog poo, the smell pretty much rejects it from going in our mouths even if we didn't know how it tasted! Which I hope you don't.

So, change this theory to artificially sweetened products; our body knows glucose is good. It can use it as energy, and the brain and red blood cells need it to function. When we trick our body into thinking glucose is on its way with a sweet taste on the tongue, our brain immediately alerts our stomach that food is coming. The body responds by warning the pancreas that glucose is coming.

This is one of those primary metabolic responses we discussed earlier; it's a survival mechanism; when sugar comes in, insulin is released like a magic key and unlocks the cells so the body can use the energy. But wait, no sugar came in. Take diet cola, for instance; it has a sweet taste on my tongue, my brain alerts my stomach that food is coming, and my pancreas starts excreting insulin, but nothing comes. Diet cola is 0 calories; oh dear, now I have circulating insulin that is waiting for a job to do; its job is to make me go and find some glucose so it can do what I've asked it to do, so drinking the diet cola will make me hungry!

How many times have you had this happen? The same thing will happen with a dash of skimmed milk and sweetener in your tea or coffee or a lovely fruity tea; it creates this constant roller coaster of tricks the body was not designed to understand.

There are a couple of other discoveries with sweeteners that shocked me. The liver recognises that it is not glucose, so it must filter it as a toxin, forcing the liver to work harder. The other SHOCKER! A study was done on the effects of sweeteners on our gut. This discovery found that people who consumed excessive amounts of artificially sweetened drinks had mutated more genes that make us pre-disposed to storing fat.

Fruit

Fruit: I wanted to cover this as we have adopted this change for potentially the wrong reasons. I don't know any diet plan that doesn't say to eat more fruit; you will lose weight quicker!

Cast your mind back around 100 years, before Brexit was even a word! It's February, and I live in the U.K. Can I source my super blueberries locally to add to my morning Weetabix? Of course, I couldn't, or strawberries or any other fresh fruit. I might have had a bit of jam to put on my bread! But that would be it.

Our bodies struggle to process vast amounts of carbohydrates, and our fruit today is highly cultivated into big, juicy balls of sugar. If you imagine the origin of the humble apple, it was tiny and quite bitter; the wild strawberry is also small and bitter; modern agriculture and the ability to cultivate crops have had a dramatic effect on how our bodies now must work to process the amount of fruit we include in our daily diet. Morally, you know you are eating an apple, not a Mars bar, but once it hits your burning pit of acid in your stomach, it all turns to glucose; I'm afraid your body doesn't care what it looked like before it went in. The signal to the brain is the same: I have had sugar.

The five-a-day rule didn't do us any favours; there are no vitamins and minerals in unseasonal fruit that we cannot find in some good leafy green seasonal vegetables.

So, in conclusion to this so-called Health food we've been scoffing at for so many years and spending so much money on, it can make us fatter and sicker when eaten in excess!

We will delve deeper to break it down further in the fibre section.

"Eat whole foods,
buy local,
buy seasonal!
and read the actual ingredients".

11

Understanding Fibre

We are constantly told to increase our fibre intake, but nobody tells us why. Understanding the different fibre types is essential to determine what benefits increasing them may bring.

We have three different types of fibre in our food: -

Soluble Fibre
Insoluble Fibre (Roughage)
Resistant Starch

A good rule of thumb I have always worked by is anything that is soft and dissolves in boiling water generally comes under the soluble fibre banner, and anything rough doesn't dissolve in boiling water and usually comes out the same way it went in is insoluble fibre.

There are many health claims associated with increasing our soluble dietary fibre. There is not much scientific evidence to back up these claims, and it very much depends on our genetics and our gut health as to how we process them, so again, this is a case of: -

"One size does not fit all".

Some evidence from trials shows that it can help raise good cholesterol and lower blood pressure and blood glucose.

The downside is that some people struggle to process these food types, and they can have embarrassing side effects on the way through! This is down to the fact that many of them, like legumes, beans, peas, and pulses, are what we class as fermentable; when something ferments, it gives off gas, which has a very windy and often smelly side effect. You can't stand to be close to a particular member of my family after a lentil curry mentions no names; she knows who she is.

Insoluble Fibre

Insoluble Fibre plays one very vital role; it helps us to Poo; if you've ever suffered from constipation, you get every man and his dog telling you to increase fibre, but they never really tell us why it helps.

It's back to the Kit Kats and the Celery again. The Kit Kats would melt in our cup of tea. The Stringy Celery does not disappear no matter what we do to it. Well, the body works in the same way, so anything that you put in your cup of tea that is still whole and sitting in it when you've finished drinking it will get sent out a different route via the small intestine and straight to the bowel. The clever thing about increasing this type of fibre is that it makes the body work a bit harder, and we do not absorb those calories in the same way, so it can aid weight loss and help improve our metabolic responses. This can play a significant role in regulating glucose and improving our insulin sensitivity.

Some foods in this group include: -

Nuts and Seeds
Skins and Stalks of fruit and Veg
Bran

An excellent way to tell if it is insoluble is that it usually looks the same as when it went in! I know you have all seen sweetcorn go in and come back out when you have looked back at the toilet.

Resistant Starch

Resistant starch: this one still freaks me out, but it makes sense when you consider the processes.

Suppose you take the four significant white carbohydrates we all know and love: bread, potatoes, rice, and pasta. These foods are often the ones people quit when going on a diet because they think they make them gain weight immediately and bloat their tummies like they are about to give birth to a food baby. This is true in some sense of the word, but it's not the whole picture.

These foods are what we class as refined carbs. They are very absorbent, so they can be processed through our body and absorb up to three times their weight in water during digestion. This creates those two temporary problems: an instant gain on the scales and the feeling that we have just grown a 9-month-old food baby about 30 minutes after dinner! Does it last? No, not generally; the body might take a bit longer to work out where it's going, and once it converts it either to glycogen for energy or stores it as fat if our internal fridge is full, it will then release that excess water out through our kidneys, and we have a: -

"I can't stop weeing day."

Inevitably, the scales come back down, but not before we have had a little paddy and sworn never to eat bread or potatoes again.

So how does Resistant Starch help this?

When you cook food, it changes how your body processes that food. It has been the most significant evolutionary change of our time. Carrots, for instance, produce a lot of starch the more they are cooked, and mashing potatoes creates more starch; this all influences our blood glucose and, in turn, needs more insulin to be excreted to counterbalance that glucose. If you take potatoes, rice, and pasta and cook them and allow them to cool and eat them cold or reheat them, they change their structure, and the starch becomes resistant. Hence, it has a different effect on blood glucose, not creating the big spike typical with these foods, therefore not needing as much insulin to regulate the rise. It changes the way they are processed; we don't tend to get the food baby feeling or see such an effect on the scales. Bread can do the same if we freeze and toast it from frozen! The other weird one is the nation's favourite fruit, the humble banana; a yellow banana will give a direct glucose spike; the riper it is, the higher the glucose spike, but green bananas are resistant starch, so if you love bananas, green ones are best!

In conclusion, Fibre plays some critical roles, but it's not quite the diet hero it's made out to be. Don't be tricked into buying foods high in fibre, as that isn't always a good thing, and it won't instantly make you lose weight, quite the opposite in some people's cases!

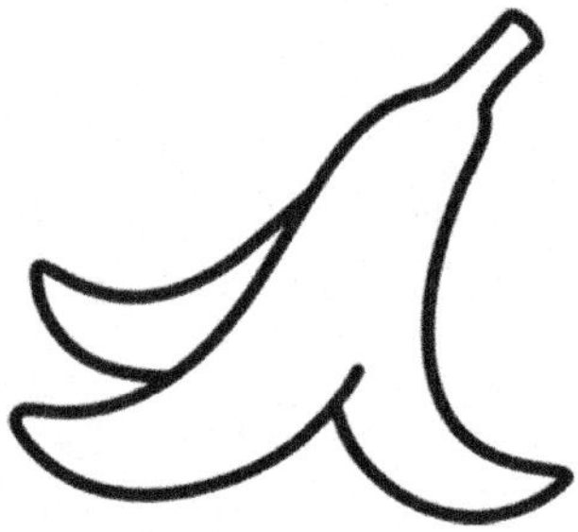

12

Hunger and Satiation Hormones

This section contains a bit of science and a few big words, but stick with me. I will simplify it as much as possible to make it easier to understand.

Most diets work on claiming they stop us from feeling hungry or that we must eat foods that keep us feeling fuller for longer; I know I indeed fell into this trap on many occasions over the years. In truth, it's all down to those pesky hormones again, the good old Metabolic Responses we have talked about throughout the book.

We do know that if we look at the three macronutrients, carbohydrates, protein, and fat, it is effortless to overeat some of them and almost impossible to eat lots of others. A good example that ***Dr Jason Fung*** talked about in one of his podcasts was sitting in the cinema with a bucket of sweet and salty popcorn in one hand and a bucket of cheese in the other. Now I know I can mindlessly munch popcorn until my jaw physically aches, I reach the un-popped bits in the bottom, and I almost break my teeth without realising, and I can still walk out the cinema and smash a KFC with gravy on the side!

Popcorn doesn't fill you up; cheese, on the other hand, as lovely as it is, we cannot eat cheese at anywhere near the same volume as we would popcorn, and our body would almost scream at us and say, for the love of God, stop with the cheese I'm done!

So, what's happening here? Why do these different Nutrients talk to us in very different ways?

In come the hormones we have touched on previously: ghrelin, or gremlin as I like to call it, and leptin, which I want to name Leprechaun purely because I think it's much easier for you to remember gremlins and leprechauns.

The hypothalamus, that clever little thermostat in our brain that controls when we start eating and stop eating, isn't smart enough on its own.

Again, this comes down to basic survival and the body's burning desire to keep us alive. Remember when we talked about homeostasis? The body likes to keep everything the same.

Ghrelin production aids the body's ability to keep everything the same; it ramps up about 20 minutes before the times that we usually eat and gives us a dig in the ribs to remind us to eat now; the weird part that shocked me was this doesn't in any way mean we are physically hungry or our body needs some energy from food at this particular time, it just means that this is when we usually eat, to keep everything ticking along the same (homeostasis), it's telling us we should now go and find some food.

Ghrelin production also tracks our weight but in strangely different ways for different people: tall, skinny, fit, active young boys have insatiable appetites because their resting metabolic rate could be upwards of 5000 calories or more, and the body knows if they do not constantly feed they will dangerously deplete their fat stores, Michael Phelps the US swimming superstar had to consume over 12000 calories a day during the Olympics to sustain his muscle mass for peak performance.

When our weight starts to increase, so does our resting metabolic rate, so again, our ghrelin ramps up, making us feel hungrier as the body is now trying to maintain this new increased weight.

This is the tricky part: When we lose weight or increase our activity with exercise, our ghrelin will rise again to replenish those fat stores and get us back to Homeostasis.

Ghrelin is fine when it behaves and works correctly, and our appestat is switched on, but other sneaky hormones tend to override it. Insulin and cortisol change how our appestat works, and then this metabolic syndrome effect happens again.

The body doesn't know what it wants when it wants it, so we give up and use the clock, our taste buds, and our eyes to determine what we put into our mouths. This, as we know, has grave effects on our growing waistline and many health implications, such as diabetes type 2.

Leptin is a very different beast. This is a considerable area for scientific research right now, and we are constantly learning more and more. Again, it's a survival hormone that kicks in to stop us from eating and eating until we pop, as we mentioned with Monty Python in his famous sketch.

We do know that children born without the ability to excrete Leptin gain weight faster than any other condition, and when injected with leptin, the weight falls off. This created a weird buzz around Leptin. We know it significantly affects weight; we don't know how to turn this to our advantage.

So here is what we do know: leptin is excreted from the fat cells, and it's a regulator that helps keep the fat stores nice and healthy and ready to protect us on a rainy day.

This is potentially why we can eat popcorn and many other yummy carbs like crisps, milk chocolate, bread, pasta, rice, etc., but we cannot physically eat vast amounts of cheese or meat as these foods are much higher in fat.

Thinking back to the low-fat phenomena that swept our nation and stuck, coupled with the shift in our macronutrient food groups to a very high percentage of carbs, this is potentially why it's been making us fatter.

I look at my Nan and Grandad (sadly, my grandad passed away recently at a very respectable 94-year-old) as good examples here. They ate only two meals daily because they didn't get up early. And that helped them live a long, healthy life, making it into their 90s!

Thinking back to the resting metabolic rates and how age affects them, they don't need much food to fill them up these days, plus my nan is only about 4 feet tall. They have always had full-fat yoghurts, cooked their potatoes in lard, fried their chips, and used a rake of real butter; they also got through more full-fat milk than a dairy cow could produce in a year! But they never got obese!

If a Dr prescribed you this diet, you would think he was stark raving mad, and it would never work, am I right?

Let's analyse it: they only eat when they are hungry. Ghrelin tracks that they don't eat early, so it doesn't come in; they eat full-fat yoghurts for brunch with full-fat milk in their coffee; leptin tracks the fat, so they don't overeat, and they have a pretty good balance of meat, potatoes and two veg cooked with plenty of fat for dinner.

They have a good balance of macronutrients, not a heavily carb-loaded diet of predominately pasta or rice that would spike glucose and create a massive insulin surge that we have been used to in our modern diets.

From this real-life example, you can see that the appestat is doing its job, leptin is tracking the fat, ghrelin knows they don't need to eat loads as they have lower resting metabolic rates; all the metabolic responses are working correctly, and the hypothalamus is working properly, signalling when to eat and when to stop eating. We are satiated, the body is happy, the fat stores look healthy, and homeostasis is maintained.

In conclusion, here in the UK, we are the meat and two-veg nation. We ate crumble and custard on Sundays and cooked our roasties in lard, which wasn't killing us! We changed to making our crumble with artificial sweetener, bought low-fat custard, and sprayed 1kcal on our roasties, and we hit the most significant health crisis of all time! It's not rocket science.

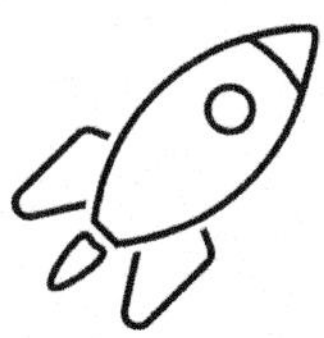

13

The Hunger Scale

The biggest objection I encounter when talking to people about losing weight is dealing with hunger. We don't like hunger. We have even invented a new word: "hangry." We think we will get dizzy or pass out if we miss breakfast!

The hunger scale is an excellent tool for making us think more about why we eat and what is happening in our bodies at these times. This makes it more relatable and makes it easier to make changes.

0 = Empty (liken this feeling to a nasty sickness bug. You know that there's nothing left feeling; even the bile came up).

1= Starving (third world poverty, actual physical starvation is horrifying to even look at on the TV, let alone experience it).

2= Hunger Pains (these are actual physical pains; I liken them to homeless people, very little food but enough to not be starving).

3= Hunger (we would start to feel actual physical hunger at around the 24-hour without food mark; weirdly, past this point, the body becomes more efficient and learns to start using its fat reserves).

4= Slight Hunger (this is between 12 and 16 hours without food; the digestive system takes 12 hours to digest what we ate last entirely, and it thanks you for a rest; the body is getting to the end of its glycogen stores and it starts to panic a bit and starts to ramp up some ghrelin to get us to replace the lost glucose. Insulin sensitivity also improves at this point as we have minimal glucose to regulate).

5 = Neutral (this is the point most of us choose to eat, usually because the clock says 8, 12, and 6. It has nothing to do with physical hunger. It is habit-forming, and ghrelin helps you stick to that schedule like clockwork. Remember, our body struggles to process too much food. It was never designed to eat three meals a day, every day).

6 = Contented (this is where we have started to listen to our appestat and are learning to push the plate away even though there are still two roast potatoes!).

7= Slightly Full (you ate the two roast spuds you didn't need, and you got up and ate the other two that were sitting on the side that didn't fit on the plate when you dished up; we eat with our eyes and we don't like waste, many of us were taught to clear our plates, please please do not instil this habit in your children it's the worst mistake parents can make to mess up a child's metabolic responses).

8= ***Full*** (you went out for a meal, you ate the man-size portion; you have a growing food baby, and the waitress appears with the dessert menu! Apparently, we have a whole other stomach for dessert!).

9 = ***Overfed*** (you ate the dessert, a cup of coffee, a glass of port, and just one more wafer-thin mint!).

10 = ***Nausea*** (just one more wafer-thin mint; this is the awful feeling when you desperately regret that last few mouthfuls, but it's too late. You find yourself walking the streets, trying to get the food down so you can breathe again. Yes, we've all done it. Christmas day springs to mind every year we say we will not do it this year!).

All joking aside, you can see that it's often not the case when we think we are starving. We need to learn to listen to the right signals.

The Brussel Sprout Test

Another one of those lightbulb moments is coming up! We have two different types of hunger. One is known as somatic hunger, and the other is limbic hunger. This is a weird concept, but it makes perfect sense when put into context.

Somatic Hunger

Somatic hunger means if we don't eat, we are at risk of damaging our health; this is true: eat to survive hunger; there have been some unbelievable stories in history where people have eaten their limbs and even eaten other people to survive, as dramatic as that sounds our bodies are again very clever they shut functions down in a particular order to allow us to reason when we need to keep ourselves alive.

Limbic Hunger

Limbic hunger, on the other hand, is what we experience most of the time; it always has an emotion attached, whether it is taste, smell, appearance, or reward; it can even create metabolic responses.

Dopamine and serotonin are potent metabolic hormones that react to pleasure and reward. Suppose your mum always rewarded you with chocolate for doing something good. In that case, your brain will connect those neuropathways and create a little signal to trigger the link between chocolate and a feeling of reward or emotional happiness.

When they tested this theory on mice, they discovered that sugar was more addictive than cocaine! It was a brutal experiment. They electrocuted the floor of the cage and placed a sugary treat in one area and cocaine in another location, and the mice were prepared to endure the physical pain of a desperate need to get a sugar fix. Still, they would not take pain for the cocaine!

If you need further proof of sugar's addictiveness, look no further than the temper tantrum of a 2-year-old who has just been refused sweets in a local supermarket. Your heart sinks for the mother, and you have an overwhelming desire to pick the child up and buy some chocolate so you can continue shopping in peace!

So, how can we use this newfound knowledge of somatic and Limbic hunger to our advantage?

This is where the Brussels sprout test comes into its own. ***Bert Herring*** must be credited for teaching me this little gem in his book ***The Power of AC Appetite Correction.***

Think of your food hell? I mean, the food that hell would have to freeze over before you would eat it. It was Brussels sprouts when I started, but I now quite like them weirdly! I then changed it to the liver, but recently, I've even started eating that, too, so I need to find a new one; I thought tripe would never find its way onto my plate, so that will do for now!

So how do you put this to the test to determine whether you have true Somatic I am going to starve hunger? Ask yourself: -

"Would I eat Tripe right now".

Replacing with your food hell for my tripe as you might love tripe!

When I do this test in my workshops, what comes up amazes me: Brussels sprouts remain at the top, closely followed by offal and fish and, weirdly, lamb, which I love. I have one lady who detests rice pudding. She believes she will never be hungry enough to eat it, so I told her I would have hers if we were stranded on a desert island and there was only rice pudding for survival!

It's a great trick to keep in your pocket to help determine what emotions we are trying to feed with food.

The other big issue here is the crafty marketing gurus of the 21st century! Those clever little people have so many tricks up their sleeves that it's frightening! The big guys in food production are now paying billions to be ahead of the game concerning marketing; this can be down to the colours of packaging, the words they use, TV adverts that talk to the reward centre of our brain, and even the specific mix of ingredients to getting that addictive I cannot live without it, limbic hunger emotions excited. We fight this battle whenever we walk into a supermarket or turn on our TV. If there's money to be made, you can guarantee they will work out how to make you buy it.

14

Do I have to exercise to lose weight?

This is a short chapter, but it is the most asked question at my workshops, so I thought it essential to include more specific details.

At the beginning of each workshop, I ask the group what they believe are the solutions to help us lose weight. You may have guessed from what we covered earlier that they always say eat less and move more.

The phenomenon is still very much what everyone believes is the key to sustained weight loss.

Sadly, this discriminates so many people with disabilities into thinking that it is not even worth them trying to lose weight if they cannot exercise. I find this sad, as that is not the case.

I once had a lady who was paralysed from the waist down attend one of my groups; she went on to lose three stone without any exercise whatsoever!

The truth is, as we discovered earlier, it's just too damn hard to lose weight through exercise alone, and as we've found, our body just doesn't like it very much and, in the name of survival, will do whatever it needs to do to prevent it.

That said, exercise does play a vital role in supporting our mental health, and I need to address it.

Serotonin is excreted during exercise. It's a potent feel-good hormone that plays a massive role in helping us regulate that nasty cortisol stress hormone, which is one perfect reason to get off the settee and out in the fresh air.

The second most crucial part is daylight. We need some Vitamin D to absorb the calcium in our food. This keeps our bones strong, and daylight is our best source of vitamin D, so that's another good reason to go outdoors.

The other great benefit of exercising is that it helps build up our melatonin and sleep pressure. To build up melatonin, we need light, so taking a long walk and getting lots of natural light has fantastic benefits to help us get a good night's sleep.

My best advice on exercise is never do it to lose weight and always: -

> *"Do something you love with people you love and laugh while you are doing it".*

Swimming and resistance exercises are scientifically proven to prolong muscle health and promote the fountain of youth.

15

The dreaded weight regain

We have discussed homeostasis and the body's reasoning for wanting everything to stay the same. This answers many of the questions behind why we lose weight, but it comes straight back again. The big thing I want to cover here is how we need to learn to think differently; if we do what we have always done, we will get what we have always got!

A wise woman once said to me: -

> *"Without change, there would be no butterflies".*

This phrase has stuck with me for many years. The biggest lesson I have learned from it during this journey is to work with the body rather than against it.

Learn why it does what it does and what makes it react the way it does; in turn, we will learn to maintain homeostasis. Life has no maintenance plan; people always ask me what I will do when I reach my goal.

my answer;

"You listen to your body, and you let it tell you what it wants."

Think back to those wild animals. They don't count calories or macros. They don't go to the gym but maintain a healthy weight!

Why We Should Ditch the Scales Forever

The humble bathroom scales, whether we love them or hate them, we have been letting them dictate to us for so many years now.

Q. Do the scales tell the whole picture?

If we look at the evidence, health professionals adopted the BMI scale as a measure of good or bad health with regards to our weight a few decades ago now; from this point on, the scales have dictated who can or cannot receive specific medical treatments under the national health service and who should be losing weight to reduce their risk of certain weight-related conditions.

The Body Mass Index is a scale that calculates a person's body mass as a ratio of height to weight. It is a simple mathematical equation; it cannot determine whether the body's mass is lean muscle tissue or dangerous visceral fat.

Every point in the BMI counts for between 5 and 6 lbs in actual body weight, so to come down 2 points, you would need to lose about 11 pounds in weight.

A scenario that shows how deceiving the scale can be is often demonstrated with rugby players. For example, for a major competition like the Six Nations, some of the props need to beef up; this can be by as much as three stone in weight, but it is pure muscle if they had a healthy BMI of 25 before the competition this would increase their BMI by around 8 points to 32 now officially putting them in the obese category, I know I wouldn't be brave enough to tell an England rugby team prop he looked clinically obese. I certainly wouldn't want to get in his way running down the pitch at full speed!

So, how does this affect our relationship with the scales?

Q. Can we convert Fat into Muscle?

This is an age-old question; I have had many answers over the years!

In short, no, that would be like turning a duck into a chicken or an apple into a pear; they are very different molecular structures in our bodies. That said, when we lose weight correctly, we can lose fat while gaining lean muscle tissue. This freaks us out regarding the numbers on the scales.

You have probably heard someone say, I know why I am not losing weight. It's because I am exercising, and muscle weighs more than fat! I would be rich if I had a pound for every time someone said that in my old slimming world group.

Sorry to burst this bubble, but not strictly; 1lb of fat and 1lb of muscle weigh the same. One can never be heavier than the other, but the muscle is much denser, so it takes up far less room in our body.

If you took a body weighing ten stone with 35% body fat and a body weighing ten stone with 25% body fat, they could be wearing completely different size clothes at the same weight.

At my current weight, I am now 17 inches smaller across my body than I was at the same weight five years ago; this is because I have reduced my fat mass by 6%. This may cause the scales to increase at times, but it's not bad; the extra muscle mass enables us to improve our resting metabolic rate, as muscle needs more energy to sustain it, so it is, winner, chicken dinner.

The easiest way to visualise this is by comparing a pound of lead to a pound of feathers. Although they both weigh the same, they are very different structurally and cannot be used to do the same job.

My top tip "ditch the scales and live a happy life without them."

Sleep

We don't spend nearly enough time asleep; this is the most overlooked tool that can aid weight loss and support our bodies to work efficiently.

Every living creature on earth sleeps, but although sleep is essential, we consider it the least important activity today.

Q. How much sleep should we be getting each night?

On average, we need around 7-9 hours of sleep every night; when I ask this in a group, it's incredible how many people react by telling me that I must be joking and that they only have around 3-4 hours if they are lucky!

In the same breath, they tell me how much they are struggling to lose weight and reel off their very long list of ailments and medications to try and fix them.

Our bodies need time to rest; it's not rocket science. This is one of the biggest things hindering weight loss and a healthy body. ***Dr Mike Mosley*** has just released a brilliant new book called ***4 Weeks to Better Sleep***; I highly recommend it if you are struggling in this area.

You will either be a night owl or an early bird; our circadian rhythm is different from person to person; if you have a night owl living with an early bird, it can cause all sorts of issues; one of you will be happy to go to bed early and be up with the larks, done the washing, made the bed and prepared the evening meal. In contrast, the night owl will want to stay up and achieve more in the evening before bed but struggle to wake up in the morning and hit snooze 15 times before even contemplating opening their eyes.

You must work out which one you are. This will help you establish a routine, get the most out of a restful night's sleep, and allow your body to rest adequately.

The two most important parts of your sleep are the beginning and the end; various apps and devices will help you avoid breaking a sleep cycle and assess how much sleep you get.

16

Why do we get fat?

We have covered a lot of ground so far. Thank you for sticking with me. I hope you have discovered many lightbulb moments along the way!

The big question we are left wondering is: -

Why do we get Fat?

I think we are confident by now that it's not the food we eat, and it's certainly not a lack of exercise or willpower!

The hormones (metabolic responses) play the most prominent role here. The question is, what can we do to control them and get them working properly?

The thing that makes me so sad is living in a society that judges overweight people; the natural assumption is that if someone is carrying excess weight, they must overeat or do little or no physical activity.

Telling an overweight person to lose weight is like telling a short person to grow two feet taller or a person who uses a wheelchair to try and walk! Don't you think we would have tried it if it was that simple?

What can we do about it?

Let's discuss some of the fundamental steps that we can implement.

Do you recall when I mentioned the participant of Indian descent on my course? He played a crucial role in altering my perspective and making me question the reasoning behind specific actions.

He had been attending my group for several months, had lost no weight to speak of, and generally laughed through much of the course; he was aware that he was at higher risk of developing type 2 diabetes due to his ethnic origin as this was something we covered on the course, he also had a strong family history, and he was significantly overweight and led a sedentary life.

I think he had resigned himself to thinking it was inevitable and there wasn't much he could do! It wasn't if it was more when?

I think back to weighing him on that day; to me, nothing had changed. I wasn't expecting much, but to my astonishment, he had lost 6 kilos, just short of 1 stone, in 5 weeks since I last saw him. This was astonishing and extremely rare in my experience working with this demographic.

I couldn't help but ask him what had changed in his life, as it just didn't add up. He told me that he was a practising Muslim, and it was Ramadan; I am not a particularly religious person and didn't know what this meant, so of course, my nose got the better of me. I wanted to know exactly how he had dropped 6 kilos in 5 weeks, knowing he didn't exercise and wasn't trying to lose weight actively.

The following conversation has had such a profound impact on my life and the lives of my immediate friends and family that I struggle to talk about it without tears coming to my eyes!

He told me that most practising Muslims during Ramadan sleep all day and eat all night; as the religious connotations dictate, they must only eat from dawn till dusk. This was summer in Gravesend, England, so dusk was around 9 pm. His problem was he worked a day job, so this eating pattern did not fit his work life. To maintain his religious beliefs, he adapted his eating schedule during Ramadan to allow him to function normally at work.

I asked him what that looked like as a daily routine; he told me that he ate a main meal at dusk around 9 pm, went to bed as usual, and didn't eat again until dusk the next day.

This planted a seed I couldn't let go of in my mind. It was eating away at me; this man had just eaten one meal and had lost 6 kilos in one month! It defied all my principles: you need to eat breakfast to kick start your metabolism, and if you don't eat, your body will go into starvation mode; our bodies are like cars. We need to fuel them to keep them running. All the basic principles I believed in were screaming at me, yet still, I couldn't put this tiny seed to bed. It was planted and already growing roots.

Hello ***DR GOOGLE,*** weirdly, when I thought about it on several occasions in my day job, people had quoted ***Mike Mosely*** to me, and even my mum had bought his book and given it to me to help the girls, but I knew best! You know that point in life where you believe nobody can teach you anything you don't already know! Yes, that was me!

One Google search led me to another Google search, and Pete was telling me he was off to bed and turning the lights out on me as I was boring company!

I found ***DR Mike Mosely's*** documentary on BBC iPlayer; I watched it twice and couldn't comprehend what he was saying was in tune with what the man in my group was doing during Ramadan, and the results were unbelievable. Dr ***Mosley*** had also lost his father from diabetes type 2-related illnesses before his time, and he didn't want to follow that same path. He reversed his risk of type 2 diabetes live on BBC TV, but still, nobody was listening enough to make a difference.

So, Google sent me on the most extensive research path I had ever been on; I stumbled from one place to another. ***Gin Stephens' Delay Don't Deny,*** closely followed by ***Dr Jason Fung and the Obesity Code*** and ***Bert Herring's Fast Five and The Power of AC***, made me realise that I had spent so much time worrying about what I was eating. I hadn't spared a single thought for when I was eating!

One of my absolute heroes in this area is ***Dr Andrew Jenkinson***. His work is groundbreaking in this field, and I recommend his books to everyone I speak to who is looking for scientifically proven answers. His book ***Why We Eat Too Much (The New Science of Appetite)*** is not a beginner's read, but if this leaves you wanting to delve deeper, I highly recommend it.

The Power of Time-Restricted Eating

The most significant lightbulb of all! I had spent my whole adult life worrying about what I was eating, or how many calories I was eating or not burning, and bingo, there was the problem staring me straight in the face; it was when

I was eating, or even more specifically, how often I was eating.

Who knew? And suddenly, all the stars aligned; rather than worrying about buying all those frankin diet foods, I could focus on making my body realise when it was hungry and feed it what it needed, and the rest would take care of itself!

It was my Nan and Grandad's diet! I was initially amazed, angry, liberated, and finally relieved!

The next day, I started a new way of eating, commonly known as the 16-8.

Time-restricted eating protocols

I had heard of the 5:2 made famous by ***Dr. Mike Mosely.*** Still, beyond that, my knowledge of time-restricted eating was minimal. 16-8 meant that I would not eat for 16 hours and then eat all my food for the day in an 8-hour window. Initially, this sounded quite a challenge. Still, I decided to jump in the next day, and in the words of ***Gin Stephens,*** I ripped the band-aid off and dived straight in.

I decided that family dinner time was necessary, and I would choose my window from 10 a.m. to 6 p.m.; this effectively meant I ate my dinner by 6 p.m. and didn't eat again until 10 a.m. the following morning.

Bizarrely, something weird happened here; the thought of doing a traditional diet always seems easy, but it's never easy as life gets in the way.

I initially thought I would die not having my chocolate chip Weetabix minis at 8 a.m. with a cup of artificially sweetened tea and lashings of skimmed milk, but to my shock and amazement, it was pretty easy!

Guess what? Nobody died when I didn't eat breakfast; what surprised me the most was after three days of scrambled egg on the yummy, seedy, thick break with butter, I realised I wasn't hungry at 10 am. This had become my new habit, and I was now only eating because it was 10 am, so slowly, over the next week, I started to push the boundaries and listen to the signals my body was giving me to eat when I wanted to eat rather than judging everything by the clock. My Appestat was working correctly for the first time, probably the first time in my adult life.

A few weeks into this new time-restricted eating regime, I spent a weekend in France with Pete. A naughty schoolgirl would surely rear her ugly head. Those who know me well will know that croissants are my arch nemesis, but remembering what I had learned from ***Gin Stephens*** and ***Delay Don't Deny***, I bought my croissant and ate it to open my eating window, which at this point was around 4 pm.

No one was more shocked than me to think I could now refrain from eating for 19 to 20 hours each day, and I was satisfied eating all my food in a 4–5-hour window. I discovered that the man in my group had inadvertently led me to what was unbeknown to me then: an eating plan referred to as one meal a day, or OMAD for short!

OMAD doesn't mean eating just one actual meal a day. It means you can open your window with a snack and enjoy a dinner of whatever you choose and even a pudding and close your window feeling satisfied that your body has what it needs for the day to make it work properly, and it will thank you for it.

The weird part of this time-restricted eating discovery was that my close friends and family wanted to play the game with me! Except for perhaps Caitlin, aka the Little Rat (4th child syndrome), as she's more commonly known in our house, she thought she would die without breakfast!

In a short space of time, 10 of us embarked on this journey. Some played it cautiously and went the 16-8 path all the way, and some just ripped that plaster right off and went for it OMAD from day 1, which made me gasp for breath!

This learning curve was fuelled by courage and personal belief, spurred on by sheer desperation! When you have run out of logical options, you are more inclined to turn to the illogical.

My girls are my driving force behind this whole study of 3. It's them and me to the end, but the ability to touch others along the way is so strong that I couldn't keep this to myself. Like ***Gin Stephens*** is spreading this message across the US, I wanted to spread this word across the UK.

Next steps

At the end of my one-day workshops and 12-week courses, people look at me and with a

"What do I do now look on their face".

One of my favourite sayings is that knowledge is power, but only if you use it. If you have read this book and made notes along the way, by now, you should be feeling quite relieved to know that it is not your fault you struggle to lose weight, and you don't have to feel guilty if you want to watch Netflix after a hard day at work rather than run 5k at the gym.

As I have said throughout the book, one size does not fit all, so it would be very wrong of me to write a so-called magic formula that will fix this. Hey, presto, we are all size zero, and our lifelong issues with food and countless failed attempts to lose weight are suddenly fixed overnight.

My advice now is to listen to your body, invest time, effort, and energy into your study of 1, and forget everything you already know about losing weight.

If the thought of time-restricted eating fills you with dread right now and you honestly think you cannot survive without breakfast, I can guarantee that your body will surprise you with how quickly it adapts. When we have been listening to broken metabolic signalling for so many years and being conditioned by the media to eat this fail-safe diet or try this fantastic new exercise regime, it is tough to see any light at the end of the tunnel.

Your body is more intelligent than you give it credit for. It will already be working out how to make you fail before you eat your first bowl of cabbage soup or hold your nose while you force down a kale smoothie that makes you want to vomit.

You can dip your toe in the water by pushing those mealtimes a little earlier in the evening and a little later in the morning, creating a 14-hour fast period with a 10-hour eating window. The next phase extends it slightly every few days until you find your sweet spot.

You may want to eat your main meal at lunchtime, or if you never eat breakfast, you need to adjust your drinks to ensure you are fasting clean.

There are no rules here; the key is to listen to what your body is telling you, refer to the tools in the book, such as the hunger scale, and ask yourself, am I starving? Or am I just used to eating at this time, so my Gremlins are playing tricks on me?

Dr Andrew Jenkinson has recently released a new book, How to Eat and Still Lose Weight. In this book, he references an analogy of your weight being like an anchor from a boat. No matter how hard we try, that boat will not move as it will always gravitate back to the anchor point. This is a powerful analogy, as we must pick up the anchor and put it down in a new pool of water.

I hope this has given you enough knowledge to want to pick up your anchor and find a new pool of water.

You have all the tools you need to start today; it won't cost you any money. It will save you money, and you do not need to buy any particular food or equipment; you need the want and the willingness to want to Learn 2 Lose.

Without change, there would be no butterflies.

Inspiration List

During my extensive experience of over two decades in the weight loss industry, I have realised that not all published studies are reliable. Certain studies have contributed to the worsening of our nation's health. As a result, my trust in sources within this industry has been limited. The following compilation consists of doctors and experts who have demonstrated the courage to challenge flawed studies and have willingly put their reputations on the line to combat the obesity epidemic. I highly recommend perusing these books to gain further insight into the matter.

Jenkinson, A. (2019). *Why We Eat (Too Much): The New Science of Appetite*. Penguin Books.

Jenkinson, A. (2024). *How to Eat (and Still Lose Weight)*. Penguin Books.

Fung, J. (2016). *The Obesity Code: Unlocking the Secrets of Weight Loss*. Greystone Books.

Fung, J. (2018). *The Diabetes Code: Prevent and Reverse Type 2 Diabetes Naturally*. Greystone Books.

Herring, B. (2014). *The Power of Appetite Correction: Boost Your Willpower, Regain Control, and Lose Weight Permanently*. AC Resources.

Herring, B. (2009). *Fast-5 Diet and the Fast-5 Lifestyle*. Fast-5.

Stephens, G. (2016). *Delay, Don't Deny: Living an Intermittent Fasting Lifestyle*. Gin Stephens.

Stephens, G. (2020). *Fast. Feast. Repeat—St.* Martin's Griffin.

Stephens, G. (2022). *28-Day Fast Start Day by Day: A Newbies Guide to Intermittent Fasting*. Hachette UK.

Taubes, G. (2011). *Why We Get Fat: And What to Do About It*. Alfred A. Knopf.

Taubes, G. (2007). *Good Calories, Bad Calories: Challenging the Conventional Wisdom on Diet, Weight Control, and Disease*. Alfred A. Knopf.

Bikman, B. D. (2020). *Why We Get Sick: The Hidden Epidemic at the Root of Most Chronic Disease – and How to Fight It*. BenBella Books.

Berry, K. D. (2017). *Lies My Doctor Told Me: Medical Myths That Can Harm Your Health*. Victory Belt Publishing.

Spector, T. (2020). *Spoon-Fed: Why Almost Everything We've Been Told About Food Is Wrong*. Jonathan Cape.

Spector, T. (2022). *Food for Life: The New Science of Eating Well*. Vintage.

Spector, T. (2015). *The Diet Myth: The Real Science Behind What We Eat*. Weidenfeld & Nicolson.

Yeo, G. (2018). *Gene Eating: The Story of Human Appetite*. Orion.

Teicholz, N. (2014). *The Big Fat Surprise: Why Butter, Meat and Cheese Belong in a Healthy Diet*. Simon & Schuster.

Mosley, M. (2019). *The Fast 800: How to Combine Rapid Weight Loss and Intermittent Fasting for Long-Term Health*. Short Books.

McCall, D. (2022). *Menopausing: The Positive Roadmap to Your Second Spring*. HQ.

Studies

The wealth of knowledge found in studies can be daunting to decipher. However, with perseverance and focus, the key studies referred to in the book can unlock the secrets to understanding the science behind the facts.

Keys, A. (1970). *Coronary Heart Disease in Seven Countries*. Harvard University Press.

Fothergill, E., Guo, J., Howard, L., Thomas, D., Sorensen, J., Harper, P., ... & Hall, K. D. (2016). Persistent metabolic adaptation 6 years after *"The Biggest Loser" competition*. *Obesity*, 24(8), 1612-1619.

Howard, B. V., Manson, J. E., Stefanick, M. L., Beresford, S. A., Frank, G., Jones, B., ... & Lasser, N. L. (2010). Low-fat dietary pattern and risk of cardiovascular disease: The Women's Health Initiative randomised controlled dietary modification trial. *Journal of the American Medical Association*, 303(6), 632-640.

Keys, A., Brozek, J., Henschel, A., Mickelsen, O., & Taylor, H. L. (1950). *The Biology of Human Starvation* (Vols. 1-2). University of Minnesota Press.

Chavarro, J.E., Rich-Edwards, J.W., Rosner, B.A., & Willett, W.C. (2007). Diet and lifestyle in the

prevention of ovulatory disorder infertility. *Obstetrics & Gynecology*, 110(5), 1050–1058.

Doe, J., Smith, A., & Johnson, R. (2022). Long-term effects of bariatric surgery on obesity and type 2 diabetes. *Journal of Bariatric Medicine*, 12(3), 45-60.

Smith, J., Jones, L., & Spector, T. (2021). The impact of genetics and environment on obesity: Findings from the TwinsUK study. *Journal of Genetic Medicine*, 10(4), 123-132.

Smith, J., Hansen, L., & Andersen, P. (2022). Weight loss in Danish twins: A comprehensive study. *Journal of Twin Studies*, 15(3), 200-210.

Feedback

What do you consider to be the three most important things you have learnt?

The way the body works with what we eat.
It is essential to allow the digestive system to rest with intermittent fasting.
How insulin affects the body

How the body works.
What is good and bad for your body?
You won't die if you don't eat for more than 4 hours.

Exercise doesn't do what you think it does.
Don't do any more fad diets.
One size does not fit all.

Low-carb is far more efficient than low-fat
Fat doesn't make you fat.
Fat is not the enemy.

How to change my eating habits
How to enjoy eating again without the guilt
You can follow elements of Keto without having to count macros.

Why diets fail.
How to look for metabolic changes
How I can start straight away without spending any money on expensive foods

How cortisol affects our decision-making
How we can put type 2 diabetes into remission with intermittent fasting
How I can improve my type 2 diabetes and reduce my medication

How important it is to eat fat.
How the body breaks down food
The difference between the types of fibre and what they do in our bodies.

Why I haven't been able to lose weight despite dieting for years.
Food is not an emotion.
How our hormones control our appetite

These are just some of the statements that I received from clients that attended either the 1-day workshop or 12-week course

About The Author

Sophie Burr has spent more than 20 years working in the weight loss industry, helping people achieve their weight loss goals. She's held various positions, including Slimming World Consultant, Herbalife Distributor, Wellness Coach, and Diabetes Educator. In 2017, Sophie lost her father to type 2 diabetes-related illnesses, and she had been struggling with her weight for most of her life. She also noticed that her two daughters were approaching similar problems. This led her to search for answers to why people find it challenging to lose weight and, more importantly, why they can't seem to keep it off.

Throughout her journey, several realisations prompted her to conduct more research and challenge everything she thought she knew about diet, nutrition, and weight loss. She uncovered answers to assist the thousands of people she had helped throughout her career. She now shares her findings in her Learn 2 Lose workshops and her first book, aimed at a broader audience.

Printed in Great Britain
by Amazon

45421736R00076